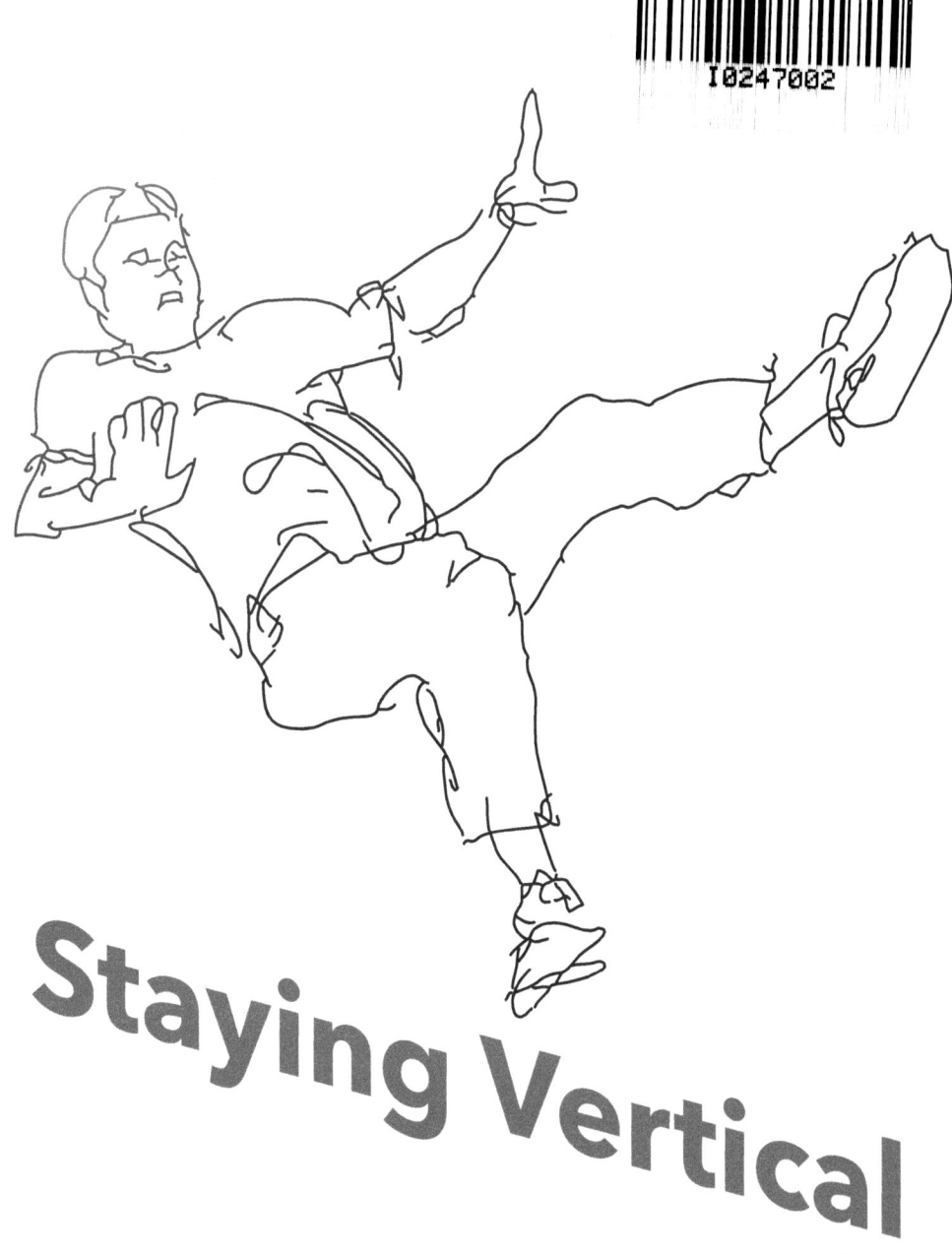

Staying Vertical
in a *hazardous* world

Arvid Osterberg

Culicidae Press
PO Box 5069
Madison, WI 53705-5069
USA
culicidaepress.com
editor@culicidaepress.com

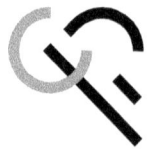

Staying Vertical In A Hazardous World
Copyright © 2024 by Arvid Osterberg. All rights reserved.

No part of this book may be reproduced in any form by electronic or mechanized means (including photocopying, recording, or information storage and retrieval) without written permission, except in the case of brief quotations embodied in critical articles and reviews.
The contents of this book were previously published with the title *We All Fall Down: Staying Vertical In A Hazardous World*.

ISBN: 978-1-68315-100-5

The publisher and author disclaim any liability arising from information or suggestions in this publication. Case studies are included for educational purposes and are based on the author's experience. To protect confidentiality all names in case studies have been changed and locations have not been identified.

Design by polytekton.com
Cover and chapter images by Arvid Osterberg

Table of Contents

Introduction and Acknowledgements   8

Chapter 1
Why You Don't Want to Fall:
The Gravity of the Situation   **12**
How to Avoid Falling   15

Chapter 2
Falling Through Life: A Persistent Danger   **24**
Falling Down and Picking Up the Pieces – My Own Story   25
Why is It That Most Falls Don't Get Much Attention?   27
Type of Missteps That Lead to Falls   28
Part of Living   29
The Older You Are, the Harder You Fall   30
The Benefits of Falling When You Are Younger   31
Not a Laughing Matter   31
Not Accidents   33
The Blame Game   33
The World View   34
The USA View   34
Standards and Codes   36
Takeaways   40

Chapter 3
Deadly Falls: Sudden Catastrophes — 42
A Hazard Waiting for Someone to Find It — 43
Why Did These Falls Result in Death? — 61
Takeaways — 62

Chapter 4
Outdoors: Paths of Unsafe Travel — 64
Sidewalks — 65
Tripping On Cracks, Hoses, and Curbs — 66
Airsteps — 73
Unstable Footing — 76
Slipping — 78
Walking Safely On Exterior Routes — 81
Takeaways — 83

Chapter 5
Entrances: Proceed at Your Own Risk — 84
Why Are Falls At Doorways So Common? — 85
Entrances and Doorways — 86
Portable Ramps and Landings — 88
Sliding Doors — 90
Takeaways — 92

Chapter 6
Indoors: Step Carefully — 94
Flooring Materials — 95
Slipping on Floors — 95
Tripping Indoors — 96
Unstable Footing and Airsteps — 99
Takeaways — 103

Chapter 7
Stairways: Tumbling to the Bottom   104
Too Many Stairway Falls   105
Stair Components and Code Requirements   106
Types of Stairway Falls   107
Abnormalities of Stairways   108
Falling Down Stairways   110
Handrails and Guardrails   115
Safe Use of Stairways   118
Takeaways   119

Chapter 8
Moving Devices: Staying Alert   120
Falling on Moving Devices   121
Elevators   121
Moving Walkways   122
Escalators   123
Using Caution on Moving Devices   123
Takeaways   124

Chapter 9
Hazardous Homes: Where Most Falls Happen   126
Too Many Falls at Home   127
Housing Sites and Driveways   128
Visitability   128
Slipping Hazards   129
Stairways   130
Reduce Falls at Home   133
Takeaways   139

Chapter 10
After You Fall: What's Next? — 140
After You Fall — 141
Living and Reliving Your Fall — 142
Should You File a Lawsuit? — 142
The Battle of the Experts — 148
Don't Fake It! — 150
Who Is Really at Fault? — 151
Takeaways — 152

Chapter 11
Reducing Your Risk and Taking Responsibility: Strategies That Work — 154
Fear of Falling — 155
Anywhere and Everywhere — 157
Stacking the Odds — 157
Learning How to Fall — 158
Getting Training — 159
Staying Fit — 160
As You Age — 161
Dogs and Cats — 163
Minimizing Distractions — 164
Taking Risks — 165
Minimizing Risk — 167
Taking Control and Responsibility — 167
Your Expectations and Risk Threshold — 169
The Benefits of a Hazardous Environment — 172
Standards and Codes Do Not Guarantee Your Safety — 173
Seeing and Observing Falling Hazards — 174
Don't Rely on Warnings — 176
Multi-Tasking While Walking and Sensory Overload — 177
Lighting — 178
Footwear — 179
Being Present — 179
Spotting Hazards — 180
Takeaways — 188

Chapter 12
Stepping Forward:
Advice for Professionals and Business Owners   **190**

State Authorities, Codes and Standards   191
Code Officials, Inspectors, and Contractors   192
Design Professionals   193
Attorneys   194
Expert Witnesses   194
Restaurants and Lodging   195
Owners, Managers, and Staff   197
Recommendations for Owners, Managers, and Staff   198
Takeaways   205

Glossary   206
References and Readings   214
Fact Sheets and Short Guides   219
Website Resources   220
About the Author   221
Index   222

Introduction and Acknowledgements

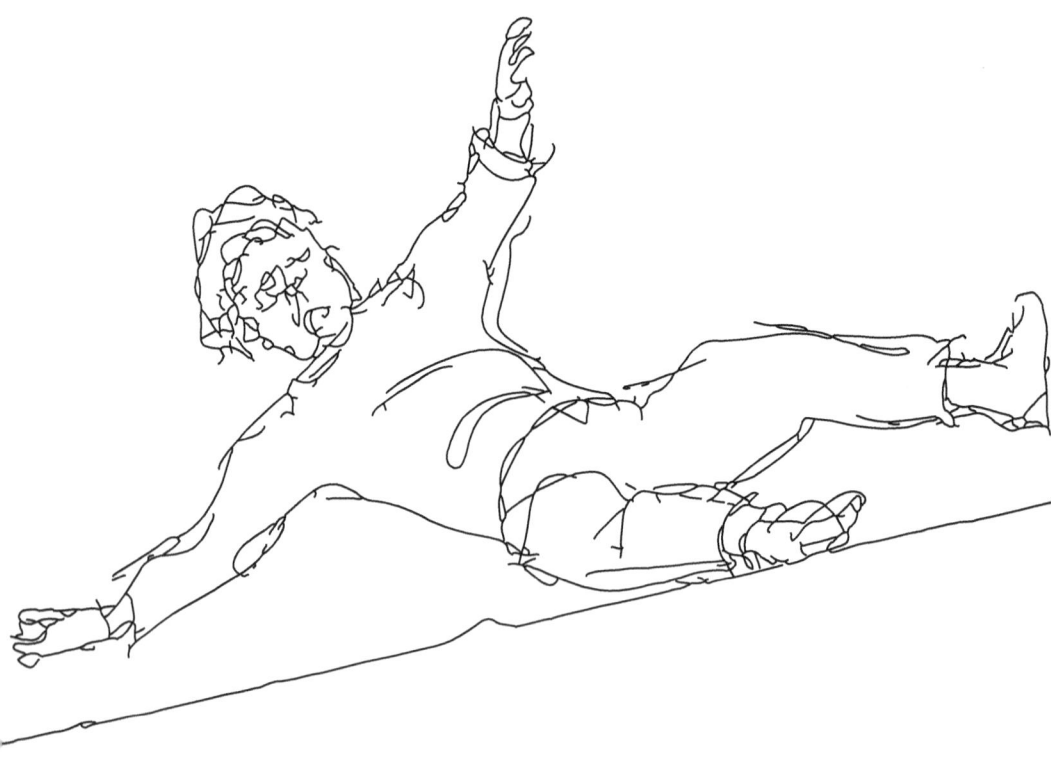

We all fall down far too many times in our lives. We accept too many falls and injuries that should have been avoided in the first place. We endure too much pain and suffering, and we experience too much regret and guilt as lives are impaired or lost forever. We spend anxious hours in hospital waiting rooms, we lose time at work and time for leisure, and we spend time in jury trials carrying out our civic duty assigning blame and financial compensation. We all pay the price for falls in the form of higher medical costs and insurance rates, expensive attorney fees and lawsuits. The planning, design, construction, and maintenance of our buildings and sites often results in hazards. Our lack of observation skills, carelessness, and unwillingness to take risk seriously only make matters worse.

Americans are often surprised to learn that falls are the third leading cause of accidental death and that more than half of all fatal falls occur in private residences. Falls result in more than 36,000 deaths every year. More than 2.8 million people are treated in emergency rooms and over 800,000 are hospitalized because of fall injuries annually. Each year over $50 billion is spent on medical costs due to falls, with the average hospitalization for a fall injury exceeding $30,000.

The information in this book can help you to; 1) prevent falling, 2) minimize falling injuries when you do fall, and 3) sensitize you to falling dangers in the built environment. It can help you to plan, design, construct, and maintain buildings and sites that are safer for everyone. It can also help you think through if there was a hazard present when you fell, if property owners were negligent for having the hazard, and if you should seek legal help to try to obtain financial compensation.

With all this in mind I began my investigations about falls in the early 1980s after I received a phone call from an attorney asking me to do an inspection where someone fell. Years of investigations followed, and in 1994 I teamed up with Professor Jeff Huston at Iowa State University (ISU) to research the subject of falls in detail. Jeff and I were both active faculty members in the Gerontology program when we first spoke about the alarming number of falls among older Americans. Jeff was developing protective hip pads to be sewn inside comfortable clothing that vulnerable seniors could wear. We decided to co-author a book on the subject with my covering safety and environmental factors, while Jeff focused on the bio-mechanics of falling. But after completing our initial research, Jeff unfortunately became seriously ill, and his life was tragically cut short. I thank ISU for supporting our initial collaborative research. In the years that followed, I completed many investigations and reports during early morning hours, on weekends and during summers. The intellectually stimulating university environment kept me motivated, and stepping back to a half-time teaching position provided time for me to finally complete this book.

I asked Steve Prater, a fellow architect, to review my completed draft. Steve's thoughtful and detailed comments motivated me to take the book to a new level, and I subsequently expanded it into its present form. I was also interested in getting an outsider's point of view on the subject, so I turned to Jim Boardman, a retired pastor. Jim is an exceptional spiritual and intellectual thinker, as well as being a professional story teller. He provided insight while helping me to reflect on what I had written. My thanks also go to the many fine attorneys I have had the pleasure to work with over the years. I have grown tremendously as a result of my interactions with them. Their knowledge of the intricacies of the law and their keen analytical skills have helped me to be more objective.

After considering various publication options, I was fortunate to be able to publish with Culicidae Press. Designer and Chief Editor Mikesch Muecke provided valuable comments, suggestions, and much needed edits as we worked through the final layout and design.

Finally, I would like to thank my wife Gayle for her tremendous and unwavering support through decades of my site inspections, reports, depositions and trials. Gayle reviewed countless drafts of portions of the book and read many sections aloud to me as she challenged me to clearly state exactly what I was really trying to say. Her patience, understanding, and empathy for me as an author, and for anyone who falls, has influenced me in many positive ways. Gayle has pushed me to a level of professionalism and clarity that I would not have achieved without her help.

Chapter 1

Why You Don't Want to Fall: The Gravity of the Situation

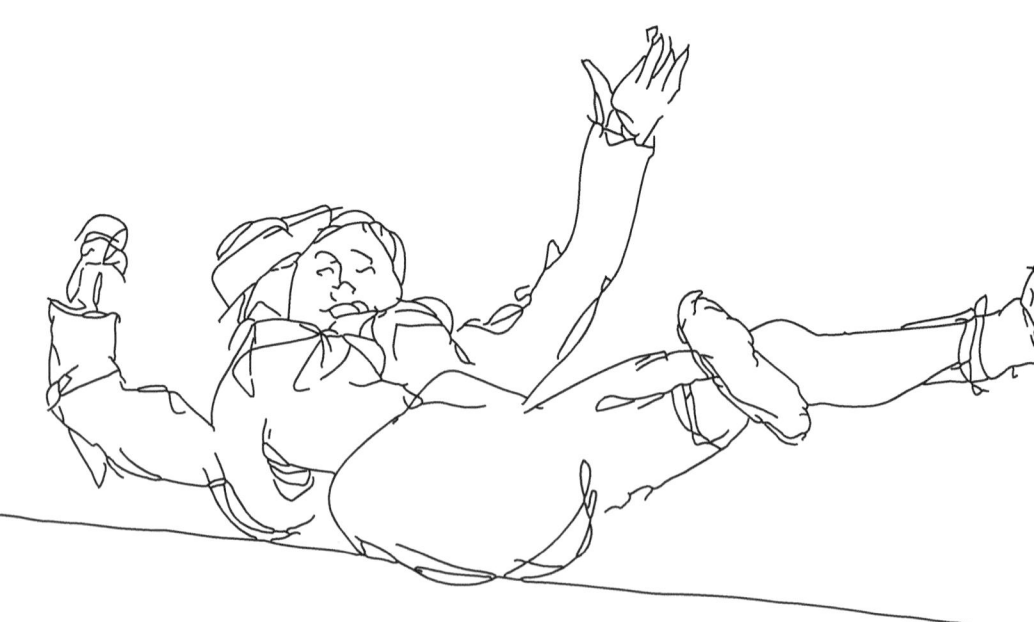

Think of all the ways we use the word fall and all the meanings it has. Probably the first thing that comes to mind is falling in love when we seem to have almost no control over what happens. We get carried away with the current and have little power to slow it down or get off. Later some people fall out of favor with the ones they love. When we are told a joke and are led up to the punch line, or when someone plays a prank on us, we fall for it. We fall victim to scams and schemes to get our money. There is also the fall guy, the person that gets blamed or falsely accused.

When we are marching with a band or a military unit, we follow certain protocols to fall in place, and to fall out. In wartime, we fall in battle, we get commands to fall back, and civilizations fall to conquerors. Our leaders fall out of power or fall from grace. There is also fall-out from radioactive particles after nuclear explosions, and there are always falling stars from both Hollywood and the sky above.

At work and in our relationships with others, we fall in line, but we also fall behind, and sometimes we fall all over ourselves. We also fall short of expectations, and sometimes we even fall flat. People fall out with each other. Our faces can communicate a lot when they fall after disappointment. Often the responsibility of a situation falls on us or falls within our duty. We also fall ill as we pass viruses from one to another. Stock prices, housing prices, even the price of meat, all rise and fall, and we are often advised to take a fallback position regarding our investments. There are also waterfalls and the season of fall when we have fall colors and fall weather. And at night darkness falls over the land.

Regardless of the many meanings of the word fall, *Staying Vertical* focuses on people actually falling from a walking, standing, or seated position due to the force of gravity.

During a typical day you probably don't think about the force of gravity. Imagine (warning, don't actually try this) that you are holding a ten-pound brick in front of your face with your elbows bent. Now imagine that you suddenly let go and drop it. Your immediate reaction is to jump out of the way, so the brick does not land on your feet. You instinctively react without thinking about it because you know the impact gravity has on the brick, making it fall fast with such force that, if it lands on a foot, it will likely break it. Now imagine you trip on a crack in the sidewalk, lose your balance and fall forward, face first. What will the force of gravity do to your ten-pound head when it hits the pavement?

When you suddenly lose your balance and fall to the surface below your feet, you are immediately reminded of the overwhelming and constant effect of gravity. As human beings we walk erect on only two feet and we have learned to adjust to a world where the force of gravity is constantly trying to pull us down. We have learned to deal with it at an early age and as adults we constantly balance ourselves against this force without giving much thought to it. When we lose our balance we instantaneously try to readjust to a stable position to avoid falling, but sometimes it is too late to correct ourselves.

As an architect and professor of architecture my interest in the subject of falls spans more than 50 years. It began in graduate school when I observed the behavior of people moving through doorways, dining halls, and public spaces to learn how well buildings actually worked for people. 8mm time-lapse film was the tool I used to record behavior. I played films back over and over again at a slow rate of speed as I questioned why doorways are difficult to move through and why people collide into each other while getting drinks in a dining hall. I asked myself why some tables were always full while others were almost always empty. I questioned why architects designed doorways the way they did and why dining halls have congested areas. I learned a great deal about human behavior and design from those early time-lapse studies, and most importantly I learned the benefits of careful observation, a skill that has helped me in my career ever since.

In the years that followed I researched housing projects, street and highway environments, older drivers and vision loss, and spatial requirements for wheelchairs. As time went by I found myself increasingly interested in what causes people to fall until I admittedly became preoccupied with the issue 25 years ago when I made the decision to write this book. Just ask my friends and family about my obsession, and they will tell you that I can't go to a grocery store or a restaurant without pointing out at least a few falling hazards. I do my best to report the most egregious hazards to the building owners and managers, but it is difficult to be assertive sometimes and, if I were to report all the hazards I notice, I would have another full-time job and would not be able to carry on a normal life.

How to Avoid Falling

There are many ways to fall and many contributing causes. The following examples illustrate the point. Each example is followed by an alternative scenario with one or two small differences to show how falls can be avoided.

Tripping on a sidewalk

You are trying to keep pace with a friend who likes to walk faster than you do. Not surprisingly, she talks fast, too, so you are also trying to understand what she is saying. You don't notice that the concrete walk has shifted and that there is a tripping hazard in front of you. Even though the raised section is only up 0.5in. (12.7mm), the toe of your shoe catches on it. How unlucky. It happens so fast that you fall on your face and within an hour it is black and blue. Your left eye is frozen shut from the swelling, your lip is a mess and you are suffering from a mild concussion. But what hurts most is your pride. You are embarrassed by your appearance and after seeing your doctor you stay home for weeks while you heal.

How not to trip and fall on a sidewalk
You realize that you should not be walking at the same pace your friend is walking, so you tell her to walk ahead if she wants to but that you need to go slower. She walks ahead because she doesn't want to be late for her appointment. You continue to walk at your own comfortable pace. You have trained yourself to glance down at the walking surface every few steps to watch out for hazards. You see a crack ahead that might be a tripping hazard, so you cautiously step over it, avoiding a trip and fall.

Slipping on ice
It is 40° F (4.44° C) outside and well above freezing, so you assume it is safe to walk through a puddle of water in your path. You thought you were being extra careful, but you slipped anyway. You have no way of knowing that there is actually a slippery ice patch underneath the puddle. You slip, fall backwards, hit your head on the pavement and suffer a concussion. You ask yourself, how could there be ice under a puddle? Ice is supposed to form on top, isn't it? Then you realize that a layer of ice probably formed in a depression in the blacktop the night before and then during the day when the temperature got above freezing, snow melted and water spilled over ice that was in the shade and did not completely melt.

How not to slip and fall on ice
You realize that you should be less trusting of what your eyes see. You are aware that it is still winter, and there is a possibility of slipping so you take baby steps and walk very slowly through the puddle, or better yet, you walk around it.

Tipping over an electric scooter
You are traveling along a sidewalk at a good clip in your electric scooter. You see a driveway intersecting the sidewalk ahead, but you don't slow down. When you cross over the driveway you encounter a severe cross-slope perpendicular to your path of travel that causes you to lose control and tip over. You hit your good arm on the pavement, and are laid up for months while suffering severe pain and bruising.

> How not to tip over an electric scooter
> You have trained yourself not to drive too fast for the conditions, so you slow down when you see a driveway ahead. You successfully negotiate the cross-slope at a slower speed with a better approach angle.

Tripping at a doorway
You walk through a doorway to a store in an old building downtown, but you are in a hurry and are hyped-up on coffee. You neglect to look down at the wood threshold at the bottom of the doorway and the toe of your shoe catches on it, so you trip and stumble forward. You instinctively stretch your arms and hands out ahead of you and suffer multiple fractures as you hit the floor.

> How not to trip and fall at a doorway
> You remember that caffeine is actually a drug, and although it helps you stay alert, too much caffeine makes you jumpy and affects your behavior. You decide to forgo the extra cup of coffee, and since you have trained yourself to watch out for high thresholds at doorways, you see the hazard and step over it.

Stepping into space
You are in a clothing store in an old building on Main Street. You didn't realize it when you walked into the store but there is a large interior space that extends into what use to be two separate businesses with two separate entrances. When the two spaces were merged together, open doorways were installed between them. But as you walk through one of the doorways you are looking ahead to the clothing on a display rack

and do not notice that the floor slopes down a few inches into the other space. When you do not recognize the change in floor level you step into space, fall forward, and break your wrist.

How not to step into space
You continually watch out for falling hazards, including sloped surfaces, everywhere you go. When you see the clothing on the display rack you are also aware of the fact that you are walking through a doorway to get there, so you look down and see the sloped floor. You are able to walk through the doorway without losing your footing.

Slipping in a grocery store
You chose the shortest checkout aisle with no waiting. That turns out to be a mistake because you do not notice the spilled water on the floor. The next thing you know you are lying on the floor and people are looming over you asking if you are ok. You instinctively say, "I think so," but a few moments later, as the shock wears off, you realize that you broke your elbow when it hit the counter on your way down to the floor.

How not to slip and fall in a grocery store
You periodically glance down at the floor as you walk. You see what looks like a wet area on the floor, so you stop in your tracks. You tell the sales attendant who calls for help to barricade the area and clean up the spill. You patiently wait in line in a different check out aisle.

Falling in a dimly lit restaurant
You are meeting your friends for lunch on a bright sunny day. The snow covered ground makes it even brighter outside. When you arrive at the restaurant and walk inside it is crowded with people and you can't see much of anything including the small child who is standing in front of you, so you bump into him, stumble forward, and fall onto the floor. You put your hand out to break your fall, but you break your wrist and dislocate your shoulder instead.

How not to fall in a dimly lit restaurant
You enter the restaurant and realize you cannot see very well. You decide to stand still inside the doorway to let your eyes adjust. After three or four minutes you can see better, so you walk over to the sign-in area.

Falling down basement stairs
You are watching a video on your phone while walking down your steep basement stairs. You know it is a bad idea, but you have gotten away with it before. You over-step the bottom stair even though you know it is there and you fall into the wall and hit your face. You break both your nose and your smart phone as a result.

How not to fall down basement stairs
You pledge to yourself not to use your phone while walking on stairs. You are aware of the fact that your stairway is steep, so you use the handrail and walk down slowly, making sure that most of your shoe lands firmly on each stair tread. You pay special attention to the bottom of the stairway where many falls occur, and you make it to the bottom without incident.

Falling down a dark stairway
After dark you start down the stairway in your house but can't turn on the light because the only switch is at the bottom of the stairway. You do not see the magazine on the stairs and step on it. The magazine slips out from under your foot and you fall down to the bottom of the stairway, breaking your shoulder in the process.

How not to fall down a dark stairway
You replace the light at the bottom of the stairs with a brighter one and have lighted three-way switches installed, which allows you to see the switches in the dark and turn them on and off at both the top and bottom of the stairway. You make sure to always turn the light on before starting down the stairway, and you never leave items such as magazines or books on the stairs.

Tumbling down a stairway

You put a stack of clothing at the top of the stairs to remind you to take it down the next time you go downstairs. But the next time you go downstairs you are in a hurry, so you step around the pile. It might have worked out except for the fact that you over-step the top stair. You tumble down to the bottom and break your arm and wrist while trying to catch yourself.

How not to tumble down a stairway

You resolve to never put anything near or on the stairs. You buy a basket with a handle to put things in so you can safely carry things up and down stairs with one hand while holding onto the handrail with your other hand. You leave the basket in a safe place off to the side and not in the path to the stairs.

Falling while carrying a box up a stairway

You are carrying a large cardboard box full of items up your stairway. Because you don't see the edge of the stairs you under-step a stair and don't get good footing. You lose your balance and fall backwards, bouncing around until you land squarely on your bottom, breaking your tailbone and bruising your hip in the process.

How not to fall while carrying a box up a stairway

You are about to go upstairs with the box when your little voice calls out to you saying, "wait a minute, you know better than this." You realize that carrying a large box will both block your view and prevent you from using the handrail. You wisely put the box down, take everything out of the box, and take three trips with smaller loads while using the handrail.

Stumbling on loose carpeting

You know the floor in your living room is covered with loose carpeting, so you walk slowly. But this time your foot tangles up on the loose carpeting and you fall to the floor and break two ribs as your chest hits the corner of a coffee table.

How not to stumble on loose carpeting
You recognize that the carpet in your living room is loose, so you hire a carpet installer to securely fasten it down. You move your coffee table out of the path. You avoid falling and breaking two ribs.

Slipping and falling in a bathroom
You slip as you step out of your tub-shower, fall on the floor and break your wrist.

How not to slip and fall in the bathroom
You realize that wet plus smooth equals disaster. You remodel your bathroom and install a walk-in shower with non-slip surfaces. You have grab bars professionally installed in appropriate locations. You make sure there are no towel bars in locations where grab bars should be. You always hold on to a grab bar when getting in and out of your shower.

These examples illustrate how cautious behavior, being able to observe hazards before encountering them, and eliminating hazards can all substantially reduce your chances of falling.

This book is different from many others on the subject in that I instruct you on how to become less likely to fall, and less likely to be injured when you do fall. You will learn how to sharpen your observation skills and raise your overall awareness of falling hazards, and to pick up on subtle—and not so subtle—visual cues to identify and safely negotiate falling hazards. You will learn how to eliminate falling hazards where you live and as you age. Advice is provided for homeowners and business owners, design professionals, building inspectors, and maintenance crews to help them identify and eliminate falling dangers.

A series of case studies distilled from forty plus years as an expert working on fall investigations will illustrate how various design, construction, maintenance, and human behavior factors make a difference. Understanding how these factors combine and interact with each other will help you to consciously observe and navigate various falling hazards so you can prevent serious injuries, and maybe even save your life.

Most importantly, you will develop a state of mind to increase your awareness of your surroundings, and to take responsibility for your own behavior in order to stay safe in an upright position. And if you still do slip on ice, or trip on a sidewalk, or step into space, you will improve your odds of a safe landing by applying what you learn from reading this book.

Chapter 2

Falling Through Life: A Persistent Danger

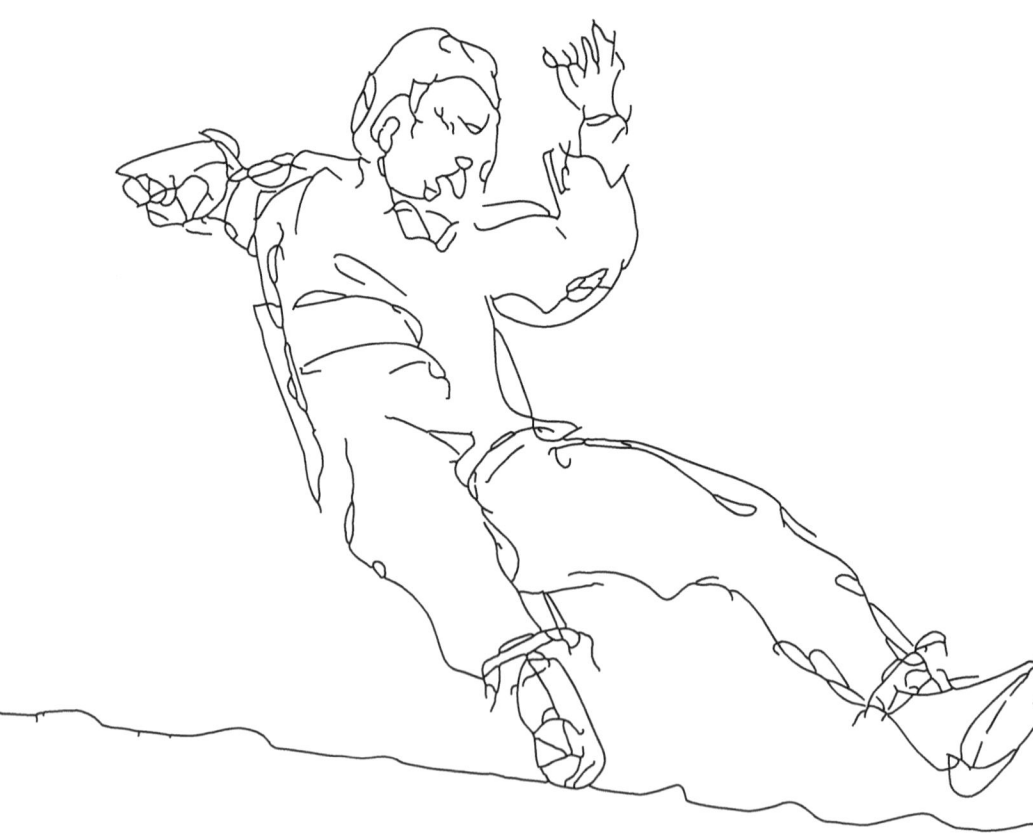

Falling Down and Picking Up the Pieces - My Own Story

Recently I woke up from a dream about falling and began recalling actual life events. As I lay in bed I remembered when I was six years old and was running up the limestone walk to the front door of our house to tell my parents something, but I lost that thought forever when I tripped on one of the rough protruding stone edges. When I fell my forehead came down hard on the front edge of the concrete stoop, and I immediately started bleeding profusely. I screamed and my mother came running out from the kitchen. She rushed me to the emergency room where I received numerous stitches. I have recalled that traumatic event many times over the years, remembering the blood and the stitches, but not much else. This time while lying in bed half awake, I came to the realization that I likely had a concussion and traumatic brain injury when my head hit the concrete fast and hard.

As I laid still in my deeply relaxed state I began to see a pattern emerge. I thought to myself that this explains a lot of things about my life for which I never had a good explanation before, like when I was in the second grade and I could only read one word at a time and not phrases or sentences like the other kids. Fortunately my teacher alerted my parents about my problem and arranged for me to have Saturday morning tutoring sessions with Miss Withrow, otherwise I might have never learned how to read at all. And then there were the eighth-grade classes for the slow learners. That is when I learned to stay in the background and became an 'observer' of life rather than an active participant in it. This led to four long and lonely years in an introverted dream state (better known as high school) where I struggled through math and science courses and learned to cope by being a quiet, reserved teenager who kept to himself. I was always the good kid who did not make waves or cause trouble. What would my personality have been like if I had not fallen and not had that concussion? Maybe it would have been different, and maybe not. I will never know for sure. I guess in some ways I am still recovering from that fall since it only took me sixty more years and a vivid dream to put two and two together and realize that I likely suffered a concussion rather than simply fell and cut my forehead.

I must have learned to compensate for my learning difficulties at some point, because I eventually graduated, became a licensed architect, worked for architectural firms, and earned a doctorate while pursuing my teaching career.

When I think back over my lifetime, I realize how many times I have actually fallen: off of tricycles, bicycles, two Segways, a surf board, a jet ski, a canoe, snow skis, and multiple snow sleds. During backyard and intermural games I've fallen while ice skating and roller skating, and when playing baseball, football, basketball, volleyball, and badminton. I've also fallen many times while trying to catch a Frisbee. I've fallen off of dirt piles, on wet leaves, on snow- and ice-covered sidewalks, driveways, parking lots, stairs, and decks. I've fallen off of foot stools, chairs, sofas, and even off an upper sleeping loft on the Gripsholm ocean liner while crossing the Atlantic.

Recently I estimated how many falls I have had over my lifetime and came up with at least 500, including 200 as a toddler, 100 as a child,

100 as a teenager, and then about 150 as an adult between the ages of 20 and 70. There has been a trend to fall less and less often as I have gotten older, especially during the past few years. It seems that over time I have learned to be more cautious, to listen to my little voice, and to stay within my limits. I know this is the case because of all the near misses or close calls I have had when I slipped, tripped, or miss-stepped but was able to recover without actually falling. I have come to appreciate that the various falls I have had in my lifetime, especially those that resulted in painful broken bone injuries, have given me empathy for other people who have fallen and suffered injury.

Why is It That Most Falls Don't Get Much Attention?

Falls from low heights are a major cause of injury, pain, suffering, and death in our society. Yet the majority of falls do not result in serious injury or hospitalizations. Can you train yourself to recognize falling hazards before you encounter them to reduce your chances of falling? Can you learn how to fall safely without being injured? The answer to both these questions is yes, as you will learn throughout this book.

Little attention has been paid to the problem of falls compared to vehicular accidents. The auto industry has improved the safety of vehicles exponentially over the past several decades, while fall prevention has received comparatively little attention. Car accidents get media coverage and public pressure, but deaths from falls go largely unnoticed, except by the people who fall and their family and friends. You are probably like most people who think "it won't happen to me," but it really hits home when it does happen to you.

Occasionally you see on the nightly news that a famous person has died from a fall. But if you only hear these stories intermittently, you tend to forget about them quickly. People are dying from falls every day, just one at a time. If you search the internet for famous people who have died from falls, you will be amazed at what you find. Ann Davis, who played Alice on the Brady Bunch, died after falling in her bathtub. Robert Culp, who starred in the TV series 'I Spy' died after falling in his home. Dr. Atkins, author of weight loss books, died from head injuries after he fell near his office. Author Kurt Vonnegut died after suffering brain injuries from a fall in his home. The list goes on. Then if you search for famous people who have fallen, but survived, the list is very long. It includes people of every age, athletes, musicians, politicians, and people from all walks of life.

Type of Missteps That Lead to Falls

Falls happen suddenly as a result of a loss of balance. Once a person begins to fall, gravity continues to work. If there is nothing to stop the fall or interfere with it, a person can fall 16 ft. (4.87m) in one second. So even if you only fall to the floor or ground, it can happen in an instant. This allows you almost no time to react or take action to avoid falling, once you start to fall. Although it is common to refer to a fall as a "slip and fall," in my experience most falls are not caused by slipping.

Fall expert Jake Pauls refers to six common types of missteps that can result in a fall as; a trip, a slip, unstable footing, an airstep, an over-step, and a heel-scuff. A seventh type of misstep is known as an under-step. I have drafted my own working definitions of each of these terms as follows, based in part on Jake Pauls' definitions. (Pauls, 2001)

A trip typically happens when the toe of your shoe catches on something, like a crack in a sidewalk or an unnoticed step, or an obstacle on the floor. If your upper body keeps moving forward you may lose your balance and fall. Falls caused by trips usually result in falling forward, and both head injuries and broken bones are a common result.

A slip happens when there is not enough friction, or slip resistance, between the bottom of your foot or footwear and the walking surface under your foot. Slips are more likely when a walking surface is contaminated or wet or when snowpack, ice or black ice is present on a sidewalk, and/or when your shoes have smooth or worn-out soles. A slip often causes a fall backwards and frequently leads to head injuries and/or broken bones.

Unstable footing can occur when you unexpectedly encounter a sloped or uneven surface, and your foot does not land with adequate support. Unstable footing commonly occurs at curb ramps, at the intersections of driveways and sidewalks, and at the outer edges of walks when your foot and ankle twist over the edge.

An airstep occurs when you are not aware of a drop down in the surface ahead of you and you continue walking as if there were no level change. Airsteps often occur where there are unexpected changes in a route, such as a single step, a pothole, a section of concrete sidewalk that has settled a few inches, or at an exterior door where there is a drop down to the outside.

An over-step occurs while stepping down when part of your foot is placed too far forward on a short stair tread (the horizontal part of the stair) or a single step, platform, or other surface.

A heel-scuff occurs when the back of your shoe scuffs the riser (the vertical part of a stair). Heel scuffs are common on steep stairways that have short stair treads (the horizontal part of a stair) or tall risers.

An under-step occurs while stepping up onto a platform, a single step or stair tread when only the front part of your foot gets placed on it.

Falls are most often the result of a combination of unsafe behaviors and unsafe conditions. The exact causes of many falls are not always known, especially when there are no witnesses or surveillance videos, or when the person who falls does not survive.

Part of Living
Falling is part of life and always will be. When we are young, we fall regularly, but the ground is closer, and our bodies are rubbery and compact. We are also relaxed and limber. As teenagers we think we can do anything, so we take many chances. When we fall, we look around to see if any of our friends saw us fall because we are more concerned with embarrassment than we are with getting injured.

And in those rare cases when we do get injured, we tend to recover rather quickly.

Even when I was in my 50s, I considered it normal to slip and fall on snowpack or ice a couple of times each winter. Sometimes my pride was hurt a little, but I discovered that if I 'relaxed, tucked, and rolled', I was able to avoid injury. There were times when falling actually made my day, because my adrenalin fired up and I found myself euphoric after falling, especially when I realized I was not seriously hurt.

The Older You Are, the Harder You Fall

When you are young you don't think constantly about dying, but when you are older you are glad to see the morning light. Some people my age have stopped buying green bananas and don't stock up on canned goods anymore. The good thing is that living day to day can be more relaxing and less stressful, and higher levels of happiness are common among older people.

Falls are especially problematic for the elderly population because injuries from falls are more devastating to our increasingly fragile body parts. If you live long enough you experience the circle of life, and as an older adult you take on many of the characteristics you had as a child. With advanced age your eyesight declines, you need more light to read and write, and for your eyes to adjust from a bright exterior to a dark interior space takes considerably longer, just as it did when you were a toddler. As you age, other changes occur more gradually. Your reflexes slow, your muscles are more difficult to keep conditioned, your bones become more brittle, and you start to have balance issues.

As a result of all these changes, falls are more likely again just as they were when you were a toddler, but the big difference now is that falls from even low heights can have severe consequences. Given your height, you also have farther to fall now than you did as a short toddler.

The Benefits of Falling When You Are Younger

At some point in your life, if you are fortunate to live long enough, you are much more likely to fall again. But since you don't have that young flexible body you once had, it is more difficult to fall without getting injured. However, if you learn how to fall without hurting yourself when you are younger, you will be better prepared for injury-free falls later in life. In other words, the clumsiness that caused all that falling may finally pay off! But for those of you who were not as clumsy as I was, read on; there is hope for you too.

It is not easy to always be on the lookout for hazards and aware of the possibility of falling. I am not suggesting that you should be constantly obsessed with falling the way I am, but I do recommend that you develop better observation skills and increase your understanding of the factors that contribute to falls.

Not a Laughing Matter

In recent history falling has often been portrayed as comedy. Slapstick comedians have fallen to entertain us since the silent movie days. Funny falling is in the movies, on TV, in advertisements, in greeting cards, and all over YouTube. If you search 'people falling' on the internet you get almost four million results including a multitude of 'Funny People Falling' videos.

Recently I spent a few hours watching 'funny falling' events on YouTube and comedy TV shows, noticing that the vast majority of falls involved people who were not paying enough attention to their surrounding conditions. There was a wide variety of falls that occurred while people were goofing around or doing silly or risky stunts. But a high percentage of falls were not the result of stunts.

Many of the falls happened after ice storms when people were apparently not aware of how slippery surfaces were. Some slipped and fell on stairs while others fell on sidewalks and driveways. There were many door-camera videos of individuals slipping and falling down wet stairs and landing on the grass, a sidewalk, or a driveway. Most did not look like they were paying attention or they were preoccupied with putting on a baseball cap or looking at a cell phone.

One woman was carrying too many grocery bags up her front stairs when the toe of her flip-flop caught on the edge of a stair, causing her to trip and fall forward. Luckily for her the bags of groceries included a large supply of toilet paper that cushioned her fall.

There were several falls of people who had dogs on leashes. They were suddenly pulled off their front porches and to the ground when their pets ran off to chase other animals. There were several falls where individuals who were running got ahead of themselves, lost their balance, and fell forward. Their bodies got too far ahead of their feet, and they could not regain their balance. One man ran into and then fell over a child.

Sometimes people got tangled up in their own feet, tripping over themselves. One woman fell while descending a stairway wearing high heels. Other falls occurred when people over-stepped the edges of stairs while walking down. I was surprised to see several different incidents when people hit their heads on partially opened garage doors and fell as a result.

Falls in buildings included one where a teacher, while talking to her class, stepped backwards and twisted her ankle as her shoe caught on the carpet. She stumbled, fell backwards, knocked over a music stand, and hit a stool as she tumbled to the floor. I saw two videos of people walking into open dishwasher doors. Both fell on the doors and then onto the floor. One woman carried a tray that was blocking her view, and a man was walking backwards when he hit the edge of the open dishwasher door, fell on it, and then rolled onto the floor.

It seems natural to laugh when you see these types of falls. And it is funny to watch people fall when you know they don't get seriously injured. But the reality is that injuries and deaths from falls are a national epidemic, and our society is paying an enormous cost for falls from low heights.

Not Accidents

One could certainly refer to a fall as an accident because a fall is an unexpected and undesirable event that usually involves chance. However, in my view the term accident is more appropriate when describing auto collisions where circumstances are, at least at times, completely out of one's control. Almost all falls, on the other hand, involve human error and should therefore be thought of as avoidable and preventable. If we could eliminate the human error, a large percentage of falls would not happen, and if we could also eliminate hazards, most falls would never happen. Hazards can hide in plain sight when there is inadequate lighting, or when a person's vision is blocked. Everyone needs to be constantly looking out for hazards that might initiate a fall.

The Blame Game

When we fall, our first thought is often to blame the environment and other people, rather than ourselves. We blame the weather, the designer, the property owner, management, or maybe the maintenance crew. But the fact is that most falls are due, at least in part, to our decisions and behaviors. The built environment is not, and will never be, one hundred percent safe. Safety is a matter of degree, and there are a multitude of factors that play a part. Let us review a hypothetical example; you are on a sidewalk in front of a main street business when you fall at night on black ice that you do not see. Let us consider the possible contributing factors from both points of view, yours and the property owner's.

Your point of view is that the property owner should have recognized the unsafe condition and corrected it by applying snow melt. At a minimum, you believe that the owner should have provided a warning until the black ice hazard could be eliminated. You also believe that the lighting was not adequate, making the black ice harder for you to see.

Now consider the owner's point of view. The owner believes that you are to blame, that you should have known that the temperature was near the freezing point and that snow and ice was melting off roofs during that day and refreezing overnight. The owner also thinks that you may have been walking too fast for low-light nighttime conditions and were less aware of your surroundings than you should have been. The owner also questions whether your shoes had good grip and if you were distracted.

Considering all of this, who was negligent, you or the property owner, or both? And if the answer is both, then to what extent was it your negligence, and to what extent was it the property owner's negligence? I will be addressing these complex issues throughout the book.

The term 'negligence' is, in a legal sense, often defined as "the failure to exercise the degree of care that an ordinary person would exercise under the same circumstances." It may also be defined as "avoidance or disregard of something that one knows should be done." The individual who fell might be negligent for not having properly watched out, and an owner might be negligent for not correcting an unsafe condition.

The World View

Falls are a major public health problem and the second leading cause of accidental death worldwide. The World Health Organization (WHO) estimates that 646,000 people die from falls and almost 38 million people need medical attention after falling each year. Permanent disabilities that result from falls dramatically increase long term care and institutionalization. Young children who have inadequate adult supervision and people over 65 are especially vulnerable (WHO fact sheet). It is estimated that by 2050, 1.6 billion people (or 17% of the world population) will be over 65 years of age (US Census Bureau).

The USA View

Falls are a national epidemic and the annual cost of falls to our society is staggering. Each year more than 2.8 million people are treated in emergency departments and over 800,000 people are hospitalized because of a fall injury (Centers for Disease Control and Prevention (CDC) Website). Falls also result in more than

36,000 deaths every year (National Safety Council (NSC) Website). Americans are often surprised to learn that falls are the third leading cause of accidental death, following auto accidents and poisoning (including drug overdoses) (NSC Website). The CDC estimates that over $50 billion is spent on medical costs for treating injuries due to falls annually, and the average hospital cost for a fall injury is more than $30,000. Falls are also the leading cause of accidental death in private residences, where more than half of all fatal falls occur each year (CDC Website).

Every year more than one third of individuals over the age of 65 fall (National Institute on Aging [NIA] website). People over 65 have 2.8 million hospital emergency room visits and more than 800,000 hospitalizations due to falls annually (CDC website). Not surprisingly, the risk of falling increases with age and goes up dramatically for those over 85. Falls represent about 40% of all nursing home admissions, and 60% of nursing home residents fall each year. Over 300,000 older people are hospitalized for hip fractures every year and more than 95% of hip fractures are caused by falls (CDC website). Older people who suffer hip fractures from falls are more likely to die from complications than younger people, and those who survive often have to move to assisted living or nursing care facilities. Hospital stays from falls are often long, and the costs of medical care and rehabilitation can sometimes be astronomical. A high percentage of nursing home admissions are attributable to falls and a high percentage of nursing home residents fall each year.

Brain injury is a national epidemic, and falls and motor vehicle accidents are the two leading causes of traumatic brain injuries (TBIs). The CDC estimates that almost half of all TBI related emergency room visits, hospitalizations, and deaths are the result of falls. Over 80% of TBI emergency room visits involving people over 65 are the result of falls. Those who survive TBI often have difficulty with memory, judgement, attention, and logical thinking. Many also exhibit confused behavior, disorganization, and personality changes.

Survivors of TBI frequently have problems with movement, vision and/or hearing. Many of these conditions can result in an increased likelihood of falling again (CDC website).

Standards and Codes

Throughout this book I refer to construction industry standards and building codes. To assist the reader, I have listed and described the most cited and most important below. Construction industry standards are widely accepted norms, whereas building codes are government adopted regulations or rules that specify minimum standards for design, construction, occupancy, and maintenance of buildings to protect the health, safety, and welfare of the public.

Published industry standards and building codes become more comprehensive with each new edition. They are revised and updated on a regular basis and are used throughout the United States and the world. Complying with the latest editions will result in far fewer falling hazards. Updating industry standards and codes is a lengthy and difficult process, and they have historically been—and should be thought of—as minimums. Since standards and codes are developed by consensus, they do not always represent the preferred best practices. Instead, they represent only what the consensus of voting members agreed to. Check with your city and state authorities where you live to determine which industry standards and building codes have been formally adopted.

Unfortunately building code officials and building and housing inspectors are not generally trained, nor is it part of their job description, to advise building owners regarding safety issues related to falls, unless there are minimum code requirements that need to be met. To add to the problem, building codes do not include many of the 'common sense' recommendations stated throughout this book.

International Code Council (ICC)
The International Code Council has developed comprehensive building and construction industry codes that are used throughout

the USA and other countries. The ICC updates codes periodically (typically every three years) when new requirements are determined by consensus voting.

International Building Code (IBC) (developed and published by ICC)

The International Building Code is used throughout the USA and other countries. It includes important minimum requirements for safe paths of travel and egress routes, including doorways and stairways.

International Residential Code (IRC) (developed and published by ICC)

The International Residential Code for One- and Two-Family Dwellings is a comprehensive building code, but unfortunately the IRC has yet to be adopted in many locations throughout the country.

Life Safety Code (LSC)

The National Fire Protection Association (NFPA) has developed, and continues to update on a regular basis, the Life Safety Code. The LSC is a comprehensive code used throughout the country that includes important minimum requirements for egress routes (safe paths for inhabitants to exit buildings).

Illuminating Engineering Society (IES) Standards

The Illuminating Engineering Society of North America (IES) has developed and published recommended practices for lighting exterior and interior environments. The IES Standards are widely recognized as the leading authority for determining minimum lighting levels for specific locations and tasks.

ASTM Standards

ASTM International is a standards organization that has developed voluntary consensus technical standards that cover a wide range of products and materials. ASTM Standards have become widely recognized and accepted throughout the design, manufacturing, and construction industries. With regards to safety and falls, the ASTM

"Standard Practice for Safe Walking Surfaces" provides minimum criteria for safe walking surfaces. Other ASTM standards cover the topics of floor mats, flooring materials, and measuring slip resistance.

ANSI A117.1

The first edition of the American National Standards Institute's publication ANSI A117.1 on the topic of "Accessible and Usable Buildings and Facilities," was published in 1961. The current edition of ANSI A117.1 is a very comprehensive document.

The ADA Standards

In 1990 congress passed the Americans with Disabilities Act (ADA). Following adoption of the law, design standards were developed. The current version of the standards, known as the "Americans with Disabilities Act Standards for Accessible Design" (ADASAD) or, as commonly referred to, "the ADA Standards" are 'requirements' in all 50 states (despite being named standards).

When the United States Access Board developed the ADA Standards, they considered the safety of all individuals, including young people, old people, tall people, short people, wide people, thin people, people with cognitive difficulties, people with physical disabilities, people with limited vision or hearing, people using canes, walkers, wheelchairs, electric scooters, or other mobility devices, people pushing strollers, and all others. The ADA Standards are recognized as minimum requirements for almost all new construction, additions, and remodeling for facilities that are open to the public. The ADA Standards do not cover single family housing.

Access for Everyone

Access for Everyone is a companion resource document to the ADA Standards. The book was written by the author of this book with the help of many others. It provides basic information about the ADA Standards and building and site accessibility, but it also includes hundreds of additional recommendations based on the concept of inclusive design. Inclusive design is design for all people, that is, design that does not discriminate or disadvantage particular people or user groups. You can download a free pdf version or a MOBI version of *Access for Everyone* from Iowa State University's Facilities, Planning, and Management (publisher of the book).

Slip Resistance

Slip resistance is an important concept in understanding falls that result from slipping. Several standards and codes use terminology such as "the walking surface shall be firm, stable, and slip resistant." However, the term 'slip resistant' is often not defined. An important reality to keep in mind is that both the slip resistance of your footwear and the slip resistance of the surface you are walking on, matter.

There are industry standards regarding the slip resistance of flooring materials and there are specific procedures and methods for accurately measuring what is known as 'the coefficient of friction' of materials in controlled laboratory settings. There is an acceptable range of numbers for the coefficient of friction. For comprehensive discussions on the subjects of slip resistance and coefficient of friction refer to the References and Readings list at the end of this book.

Measuring slip resistance in the field is often difficult and unreliable. Too little slip resistance is hazardous, but too much slip resistance can also be hazardous. When I investigate a fall where someone slipped, the fact that the person slipped is typically not in dispute, and often there is surveillance video of the event.

A logical question is: was the surface the person fell on too slippery? Another question is: did the individual who slipped have footwear with adequate slip resistance? There are also issues regarding awareness and responsibility. Should the owner have been aware of the slippery condition, and should the owner have done something to correct the problem? Should the person who fell have been aware of the slippery condition, and should that person have been more cautious? Did the individual who slipped have worn-out, slippery footwear?

Case Studies
In the case studies that follow, environmental hazards and the behavior factors in various falling events are identified and discussed. My intent is to educate the reader on how various factors contribute to falling. The accounts of individual's falls are based on investigations that I have completed. However, all names have been changed and specific locations have not been identified. To the best of my ability, I have described the circumstances of each event as accurately as possible.

Takeaways
We all step up - we all step down - but too often we fail to look around
The falls I have experienced in my life have helped me develop empathy for people who have injured themselves by falling. My falls have also made me think deeply about what causes falls. Everyone falls multiple times throughout their lives, often without injury. However, too often falls result in serious injuries or death. Falls are a national and a global epidemic, and the costs, both financial and otherwise, are gargantuan. Reducing the number or falls and injuries from falls will benefit all of society by lowering medical and insurance costs, by reducing unnecessary pain and suffering, and by increasing productivity and the overall quality of life.

Chapter 3

Deadly Falls: Sudden Catastrophes

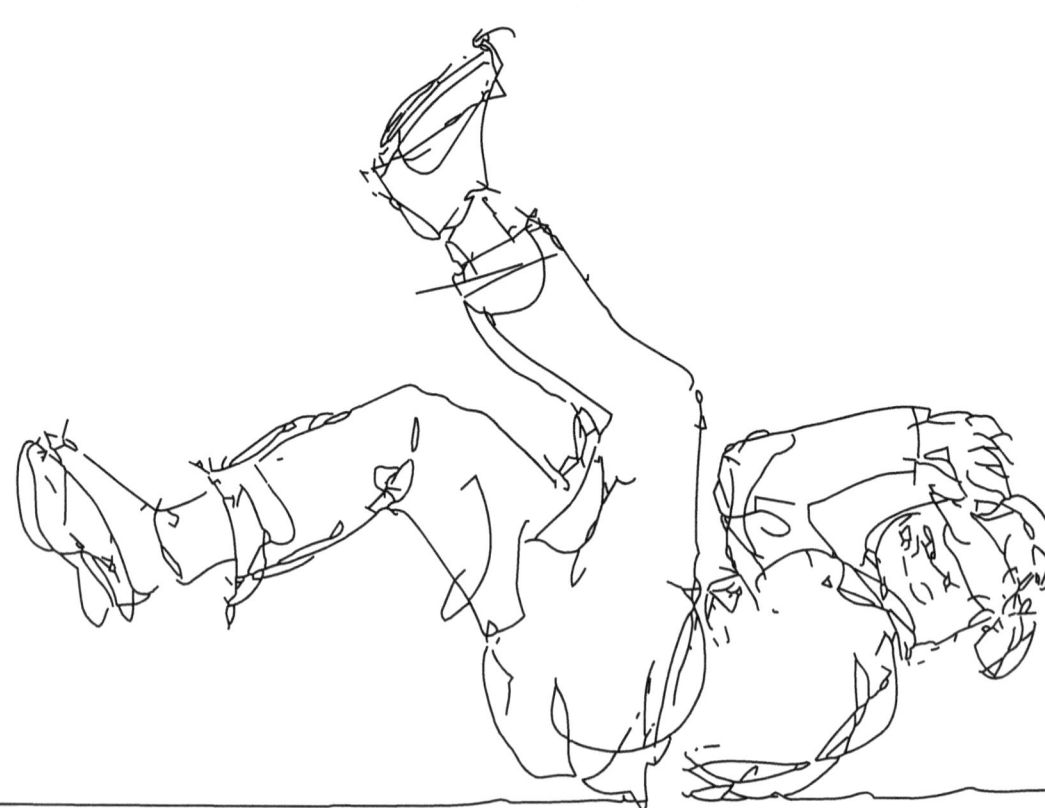

A Hazard Waiting for Someone to Find It

Many falls I have investigated over the years seemed, at first, like extremely unlikely events, but as I researched the circumstances they seemed more like hazards waiting for someone to finally come along and find them. Some of those falls resulted in death. The following case studies represent a few of the falls I have investigated that were fatal, and each case had its own unique set of circumstances. If a deadly fall had happened to a family member of yours, you would undoubtedly be asking yourself the 'what ifs'. What if he had not been drinking? What if she had not been on medication? What if he had not been texting while walking? What if the lighting had been better? What if there had been a handrail? What if the stairs had been properly constructed? What if the sidewalk had not been covered with ice? Although the following examples are simplified accounts of complex events, lessons learned from these examples can help us avoid falling in the future.

My Research Methodology

When I am contacted by an attorney representing either the plaintiff, the person(s) who files suit to seek financial compensation and/or a remedy, or the defendant, the person(s), or party(s) [building owner, company, business, etc.] who have a civil lawsuit filed against them, and asked to investigate the circumstances of a fall, it usually starts with a phone call. Following the phone call, the attorney sends me photos of the site of the incident and a description of what happened. I review the information and call the attorney to discuss the specifics of the matter. About fifteen to twenty percent of the inquires I receive either get dropped, or the attorney for the plaintiff decides not to take the case, or I decline to work on the case because it is either not in my area of expertise or I do not believe I can be of help. If the attorney does decide to retain my services, I provide a rates letter and resume. Once I agree to work on the matter, I am provided more information as it becomes available, such as accident reports, recorded statements of the plaintiff, answers to interrogatories, which are written questions by either the plaintiff or defense to establish important facts that must be answered truthfully by the other party, and depositions or sworn testimony under oath taken down in writing.

Most, but not all my investigations include a site inspection. If the site of the fall has not been altered since the fall occurred, a site inspection is usually arranged. Site inspections are often helpful because additional variables and/or safety issues become apparent. There are often inadequacies related to planning, design, or construction—such as inadequate lighting—that were not evident from examining photos and other materials.

During my site investigations I rely on both observation and physical measurements. In addition to several tape measures and straight measuring devices, I use several high-quality digital levels (of varying lengths) to measure and document slopes. When measuring lighting levels, I use a high-quality light meter that accurately records light levels down to a very low magnitude. I calibrate the digital levels and light meter frequently to assure accuracy in the field. I use a high-end digital camera, with interchangeable lenses, that has a tilting screen, allowing me to take photos with the camera flat on the ground. Over time I have found that it is better to have too many photos than not enough.

Following my site inspection, I thoroughly review my photos, measurements, slope measurements, sketches, and notes. I also review codes, standards, and other documents that are relevant to the location, before writing a report. A report for the plaintiff is typically longer and more time consuming than a report for the defense because several drafts of reports for plaintiffs are usually necessary for me to fully explain the circumstances of the fall, the unsafe conditions, and the violations of codes or standards.

A High Step

Stepping up a high step had devastating consequences for a grandmother when she went for a visit to her daughter's rental townhouse. Emma Smith had stepped up the high step many times before on previous visits. But this time her leg gave way and she fell backwards, breaking both her wrist and her hip. After surgery and months of rehabilitation and physical therapy, she died of complications from the fractured hip. Before she died, Emma filed suit against the owner of the townhouse, and following her death her daughter pursued the case. I felt anguish for Emma and her daughter for all the pain and suffering they had experienced after Emma fell.

As an expert witness for the plaintiff, I completed a site inspection before Emma passed away. My site inspection revealed three major problems with the location; the sidewalk had settled over time resulting in a 9.5in. (0.25m) step from the sidewalk to the concrete landing (the flat level platform) at the front door. The sidewalk had settled unevenly resulting in another problem: a severe cross-slope (slope perpendicular to the direction of travel), and there were no handrails (securely fastened railings used for grasping and support).

When Emma attempted to step up, maintaining her footing was more difficult because the step was unusually high and because the sidewalk and the landing were both sloping sideways. Building codes typically establish the maximum height of any stair riser (the vertical portion of the stair) as 7.0in. (0.18m) or 7.5in. (0.19m). Older building codes permitted up to 8.0in. (0.20m). However, the height of 9.5in. (0.25m) where Emma fell was excessive and unsafe, and although the step may have complied with the building code when it was originally constructed, after the sidewalk settled, the height no longer complied.

The property owner had an obligation to maintain a safe environment and when the sidewalk settled over time, the owner should have inspected the property and been aware of the situation and then should have corrected the unsafe condition. The photos I took during my site inspection was convincing evidence that the condition of the sidewalk and landing was unsafe and not 'just a little bit' out of compliance. The case went to trial and the jury awarded a substantial sum of money to Emma's estate. I have not been back to the location where Emma fell, but I assume the owner has eliminated the hazard.

A Doorway

Ken Williams went out to lunch with his wife Patricia at a local family-owned restaurant. After finishing lunch, they walked out the back door of the restaurant on their way to the parking lot. Ken was walking behind Patricia when he tripped on a high threshold at the doorway. A threshold is a metal (or sometimes wood) board at the bottom of the doorway that typically covers the joint where two different materials or surfaces come together. Ken fell forward, hit his head on the concrete and died a few hours later from his injuries.

Patricia's attorney hired me and sent me photos and measurements of the doorway and the threshold. The attorney also provided a detailed account of the circumstance of Ken's fall. Since the restaurant was in another state and there was ample documentation of the location and circumstances of the fall, the attorney decided not to have me conduct my usual site inspection.

It was clear from the photos and measurements that there was a tripping hazard at the threshold where a vertical change in level exceeded 1.0in. (25.4mm). Ken tripped and fell when the toe of his shoe caught on the threshold as he walked through a doorway. There was no warning, such as bright colored paint along the edge of the raised threshold to make the hazard easier to recognize. The toe catcher cost Ken his life. Although thousands of customers had successfully navigated the doorway before Ken tripped and fell, it was indeed an unsafe condition that was essentially a hazard waiting for someone to find it.

I wrote a report describing the unsafe threshold at the restaurant as a tripping hazard that did not comply with the ADA Standards or the building code due to the vertical change in the route that exceeded 0.5in. (12.7mm) in height. Patricia was relieved when the case settled before the scheduled trial. I would be surprised if the owner has not replaced the unsafe threshold with a low-profile threshold.

A Patio
Tyler Walsh lived in a rent-subsidized apartment building in a midwestern city. He used his walker several times a day to make his way to a patio near the front entrance of the building to have a smoke. On the day he fell, Tyler was standing on the patio and as he turned his walker to leave, the right front leg of the walker dropped off the edge of the concrete patio, causing him to fall. Once he lost his footing there was nothing to stop him from falling eight feet down an embankment. Tyler died from his injuries a short time later.

As an expert for the plaintiff, I conducted a site inspection and took measurements and photos of the location where Tyler fell. I noted that the grass area that adjoined the edge of the concrete patio was five inches below the top of the patio, making the edge of the patio hazardous. I also noted that the top of the embankment was only one foot away from the edge of the patio, and there was no guardrail to prevent someone from falling down the embankment.

A guardrail is a 42in. (1.1m) minimum high railing or wall complying with building code requirements that prevents people from falling to a lower level. Guardrails are required on the open sides of landings and porches when the height to the level below is thirty inches or more. Tyler fell eight feet to his death in a location that should have been protected with a guardrail.

I submitted a report stating my opinion that the location where Tyler fell was hazardous and did not comply with the building code because the open side of the patio did not have a guardrail. With my report the attorney was able to make a compelling argument because there were actual building code violations, known as 'negligence per se'. The case was settled before going to trial and Tyler's estate received a substantial financial settlement. A few months after the case settled, I went back to the location where Tyler had fallen and was pleased to see that a new guardrail had been installed along the edge of the patio to prevent someone else from falling in the future.

Tipping Over

Bill Smart was in his eighties and living in a nursing home. When he had a medical condition flare up the nursing staff determined that he should go to the hospital for further examination. When an emergency vehicle arrived at the front door of the building, paramedics rolled a gurney (a raised stretcher on wheels) into the building and down the hallway to his room. They loaded Bill onto the gurney, strapped him down and rolled him back down the hall and out the front door. However, as they turned the gurney around to position it to load it into the vehicle, one of the wheels caught in a crack in the concrete and the gurney flipped over onto its side. Bill's head hit the concrete and he died later from head injuries.

Bill's adult children hired an attorney who asked me to investigate. I inspected the location where the gurney tipped over and noted the size and shape of crack that caught the wheel of the gurney. It was an irregular shaped jagged crack with small stones and steel reinforcement bars exposed. Small cracks had developed in various places in the concrete and spalling had occurred when water penetrated the surface, froze and expanded, causing portions of the surface to break loose. It was evident that the owner had attempted to patch the surface, but the concrete continued to deteriorate when the patching broke loose. Although the crack was less than 1.0in. (25.4mm) deep, it had a rough surface and was deep enough to catch the wheel of the turning gurney, a device with a high center of gravity that toppled over easily when the wheel got stuck.

Patching is, at best, a temporary short-term fix that typically fails during changing weather when the patching expands and contracts at a different rate than the surrounding surface material, and when water seeps into new cracks that form between the patches and the adjoining surface. This in turn leads to more spalling. When the concrete surface has many cracks, the problem is multiplied.

All exterior concrete surfaces that are exposed to the elements are subject to deterioration over time. However, the concrete in this case appeared to be of poor quality. A common problem is when workers mix in too much water on the job site as the concrete is poured. This makes the concrete easier to work with, but also reduces its strength. Another common problem is when the concrete cures too quickly in sunny, hot weather, reducing the integrity of the material. Deterioration also occurs when too much salt is used to melt snow on new concrete.

Regardless of the cause or causes of the deterioration, the owner had a responsibility to inspect the site on a regular basis and to identify safety hazards and provide a warning, for example by spraying bright colored paint on the tripping hazards until repairs could be made. The best solution would have been to completely remove all the cracked and broken material, prepare the sub-grade surface with proper compaction, drainage and slopes, and pour new concrete. The owner should have known that the surface could not be adequately repaired with patching, that patching was not going to last, and that the solution was the complete removal and replacement of the concrete.

I wrote a report and testified at trial that the deteriorated section of concrete was unsafe and not in compliance with the ADA Standards or industry standards. A few days later I read in the newspaper that the jury's decision was for the plaintiff and the owner of the nursing home would be required to pay a substantial amount in compensation to Bill's estate. I drove past the nursing home a year after Bill's death, and the concrete surface had been removed and replaced.

Before the trial I thought to myself: who was negligent and who was responsible? Was it the emergency crew for not using proper care in turning the gurney around? Was it the owner of the nursing home for not correcting the unsafe condition? Was it the manufacturer of the gurney who designed it to be top heavy and easy to tip over? Were each of these parties responsible to various degrees? Bill, of course, was totally innocent of any negligence in this case. Perhaps this made it easier for the jury to come to their decision. The jury may also have thought that a nursing home owner should be held to a higher standard than owners of other businesses.

Getting in a Wheelchair

Jan and Fred Clemens returned to their apartment complex after shopping. There was a light rain, and it was dark when Fred drove into the parking lot and parked his van. After he parked, he took Jan's wheelchair out and placed it on the concrete sidewalk. Then he opened the passenger side door and helped her out. Jan held onto Fred's arm as they walked a few feet to the wheelchair, but when Fred attempted to assist Jan in sitting down in her wheelchair, the wheelchair slipped, and Jan fell and hit her head on the pavement. She suffered severe head injuries and died a short time later as a result of the fall.

Fred decided to sue the owner of the apartment complex. His attorney met me at the site where I inspected and photographed the site before dark. I examined the concrete surface, took slope measurements and documented the locations of the light poles. Then, after dark, I went back to the site and measured the lighting level on the concrete walking surface where Jan fell. Each of the light readings I took measured less than 0.1 foot-candles (1.09 lumens) or one tenth of one foot-candle (10.76 lumens). One foot-candle is the approximate amount of light you would get from having one candle one foot (0.3m) away from you in a dark room, so one tenth of that amount of light on a surface is more like that of a lit match, which is well below the minimum standard for safety set by the Illuminating Engineering Society of North America (IES).

The parking lot had no lights at all, and evidence showed that two of the lamp posts near the sidewalk were not working when Jan fell. In addition, the area next to the parking lot was a dark wooded area which absorbed rather than reflected any light. I also noted that there were depressions in the concrete surface where Jan fell that allowed rainwater to puddle and make the surface wet and probably slippery when she fell.

I determined that the location where Jan fell was hazardous and unsafe at the time of her fall, primarily due to inadequate lighting that was below minimum standards for safety. The case went to trial where Fred admitted that he had not fully locked the wheels on the wheelchair before helping Jan into it. Even though it was shown that the area was extremely dark, the jury found the owner to be less negligent than Fred was, and therefore Fred did not receive any financial compensation for his wife's death. The trial was in a small rural community where it was difficult for Fred's attorney to convince the jury that the owner was responsible for Jan's death. I have not been back to the apartment complex, but I think it is safe to assume that the owner has improved the lighting on the parking lot and the sidewalk surfaces.

The Edge of a Sidewalk

Sam Sanders was using his electric scooter when he encountered a curved walk with excessive cross-slope (perpendicular to the direction of travel). There was a light covering of snow when he left his apartment to catch the bus that was waiting for him in the parking lot. When Sam drove on the curved portion of sidewalk, he veered off the outer edge of the sidewalk and tumbled down the hillside, landing on rocks and hitting his head. He was rushed to the emergency room but died a few hours later. Sam's family decided to file suit against the owner of the apartment building, and I was retained by the family's attorney.

I conducted a site inspection and documented the cross-slope in various locations on the walking surface. I learned that Sam had traveled on the curved walk many times before since it was the only route for him to use to get from his wheelchair-accessible apartment on the back side of the building to the parking lot in front. It was an older apartment building that had a stairway leading up to the front door, so he had no choice but to traverse the curved sidewalk daily to get to his apartment. I noted that the most severe cross-slope was on the curved portion of the walk and that it leaned to the outside towards a steep grassy hillside that dropped way down to a street below.

Because the walking surface was curved and had an excessive cross-slope that leaned to the outside of the curve, the situation was very hazardous, especially when the surface was covered with snow. To visualize this situation, imagine driving your car on a curved exit ramp of a highway at a cloverleaf style interchange. Since the curved section of roadway slopes towards the inside of the curve it helps resist the natural tendency and momentum of the vehicle to drive off the outside edge of the curve. The banking of the curved section of roadway helps you stay on your path and makes the situation safer by keeping you from driving into the ditch. Even with the proper slope, occasionally you will see an overturned vehicle that drove too fast going into the curve.

Now imagine a curved sidewalk that slopes the opposite way towards the outside of the curve. In this situation the outside edge of the curve is also the lowest portion of the sidewalk. Now visualize a hillside that also slopes down and away from the curved edge of the sidewalk. The combination of the excessive cross-slope in the wrong direction—opposite of the curved exit on the roadway—and the hillside sloped down and away from the outside of the curve, and you have a recipe for disaster.

An excessive cross-slope makes the pull towards the low side very strong, even when you are on a straight section of walk. If you have strong arms and are using a manual wheelchair it helps to use your hand and arm strength to resist the pull to one side. This is a phenomenon you become very aware of when you first use a manual wheelchair on walking surfaces with cross-slope. When you are using a motorized wheelchair or electric scooter, it is easy to go too fast and the tendency to veer off the path is great.

This explains why design and construction standards, including the ADA Standards, prohibit cross-slopes on accessible routes that exceed 2%. The problem, however, is that this standard is frequently not adhered to, and many routes have cross-slopes that exceed 2%.

My report documented the excessive cross-slope on the curved walkway, and I provided a detailed explanation of why the situation was unsafe. Shortly before the trial, for reasons I do not fully understand, the judge ruled that I would not be allowed to state my opinion that the sidewalk was unsafe and that I could not refer to the ADA or any violations of the ADA Standards during the trial. The judge ruled that I would only be allowed to testify that I had conducted a site inspection and to state my cross-slope measurements. The plaintiff's attorney decided to have me testify at trial anyway, despite the judge's rulings.

A combination of factors lead to Sam's tragic death, and the jury had many questions to address. Did Sam drive his motorized scooter too fast or recklessly? Was the owner of the apartment building negligent for not rebuilding the portion of sidewalk with the excessive cross-slope? Was the owner negligent for not removing the snow in a timely manner? Should the owner have installed a guardrail or fence?

During the trial, evidence was presented that another resident who was also using an electric scooter had previously driven off of the same curved sidewalk and tumbled down the same hillside. He was shaken up and bruised but survived his fall without serious injuries.

To my surprise the jury found for the defense and Sam's family received no financial compensation. The plaintiff's attorney spoke to jurors after the trial who told him they did not understand why the expert (referring to me) only spoke about his slope measurements but did not testify about the condition being unsafe or not in compliance with standards. But of course, I was not allowed to speak to those issues due to the judge's ruling. However, the jury did not know anything about the judge's ruling. The plaintiff's attorney wanted to appeal and request a new trial, but Sam's family decided they had been through enough and did not want to go through the ordeal of another trial.

Taking a case to trial can be very stressful and traumatic for plaintiffs and their families. Defense attorneys often play hard ball and try to place the blame on the person who fell, even when that individual is no longer alive to explain what actually happened. I thought that common sense would prevail with the jury, but it didn't appear to. However, since I was not permitted to be present during the entire trial, I did not hear all the evidence that was presented to the jury.

It was satisfying for me to learn that after the trial a fence was installed near the edge of the sidewalk to prevent someone else from falling down the hillside where Sam had suffered his fatal fall. Even when the defense wins at trial and is not found to be negligent, the building owner is wise to make improvements to eliminate a falling hazard.

Stairways

Jim Clover went to a party in an apartment on the second floor in a building on Main Street. The building had a business on the first floor and an apartment above on the second floor, which is typical in many Main Street buildings. When Jim left the apartment, he fell down a stairway. There were no witnesses to the fall, and Jim was found a short time later at the bottom of a stairway. His body lodged in front of a door that opened onto Main Street. He suffered serious head injuries, went into a coma, and died several days later after an expensive hospital stay. A few months after the incident his children brought suit against the owner of the building.

I was hired by the attorney representing Jim's family. When I inspected the stairway, I observed and noted several code violations, irregularities, and unsafe conditions. The primary unsafe condition was to have only one light at the top of the stairs that was operated by a switch, rather than remaining on at all times. To make matters worse, the light bulb was burned out when Jim fell. The second unsafe condition was to have only one handrail in the stairway, and it was loose and did not extend to the top of the stairway. This made it necessary for anyone descending the stairway to lean down into the stairway in order to grab hold of the end of a loose handrail. The third unsafe condition was the excessive wear and dirt on the wood stair treads that made the steps slippery.

There was evidence that Jim had been drinking at the party and was legally drunk when he fell down the stairs. But the stairway was also unsafe. So, the question was, did any of these safety issues contribute to Jim's fall, and if so, to what extent? Common sense would suggest that, even though Jim was drunk, insufficient lighting was a contributing cause. I wrote a report stating that a dark stairway with worn, slippery stair treads, and a loose handrail that did not extend to the top of the stairway, is not a safe stairway to exit a building. I also cited relevant building code and life safety code violations. The case was settled before going to trial, and Jim's family was pleased with the financial compensation they received, but of course they would have preferred to have Jim back with them. Once a life is lost to a fall, that life is gone forever.

I hope the building owner has installed a light in the stairway that stays on all night and cannot be turned off by residents.

Hugh Sauer stopped by his daughter Carol's duplex apartment to deliver a package to her. The building had an entrance from the street and another entrance from the back where the driveway and garages were located. The postal delivery people and other first-time visitors used the front door, but family and friends always used the back entrance. The back entrance had an interior landing with a door on the right opening to one apartment, and a door on the left opening to the other apartment. If you entered the outside door and walked straight ahead you would walk down an open stairway—there was no door or railing present at the top of the stairs—to the basement where the laundry and storage for both apartments were located.

Carol lived in the apartment on the right, so when Hugh entered the building he turned to his right and knocked on her door. Carol opened the door and greeted her father while he stood on the landing outside her apartment. As Hugh stood there with the open stairway to his left someone came out of the other apartment door behind him, causing Hugh to instinctively move over a step to make room for that person to go outside. But when he stepped out of the way, his left foot went over the top edge of the open stairway and he suffered a fatal fall to the bottom of the stairway.

Carol filed suit against the building owner, and her attorney requested my services. Carol's attorney was there to meet me when I arrived to inspect the location where Hugh had fallen. We went into Carol's apartment and spoke with her concerning the circumstances of her father's fatal fall. My inspection and measurements revealed that the landing at the top of the stairs was very small and did not extend to the edge of the doorway (or beyond the edge of the doorway) as required by the building code.

The building had started out as a single-family ranch style house but had been converted into two apartments—a duplex—several years before Hugh fell. However, when the house was converted into a duplex, the owner apparently tried to keep construction cost low, and that resulted in the small landing at the top of the open stairway where three doors (the entrance door to the building and the interior doors to each apartment) were all in a close proximity to the top of the open stairway. Because the landing was small, there was not adequate room to stand in front of the doorway to the apartment without Hugh's left foot being perilously close to the top edge of the stairway. Adding to the problem was the fact that the entrance door to the building swung into the space, so when Hugh stepped aside to make room for the other person to get around him, he unintentionally stepped over the edge and into space, and there was nothing within reach for him to hold onto to stop his fall.

Open stairways near doorways can be very hazardous. The International Residential Code (IRC) includes detailed requirements for stairways, landings and doorways in residential construction, and the location where Hugh fell would not have complied with IRC requirements. However, the vast majority of existing housing, including Carol's duplex, were constructed before the IRC was written, and even if her duplex had been newly constructed, it might not have made a difference, since many states and/or municipalities still have not adopted the IRC.

I wrote a report describing the unsafe conditions at the landing at the top of the open stairway and also cited unsafe conditions in the stairway itself. However, since I could not cite specific building code violations, Carol was fortunate to be able to settle the case for an undisclosed amount before the scheduled trial. Although I do not know for sure, I assume that the owner of the duplex has installed a gate at the top of the open stairway.

When I was writing my report for Carol's attorney, I recalled that I had investigated a very similar case earlier. However, that time I was working for the defense. In that incident Nancy Cain, the plaintiff, was sitting and talking with a group of friends in her neighbor's back yard. When she needed to use the bathroom she was told to go in the house, turn right and go through the door to the kitchen to get to the bathroom. However, when she entered the back door of the house and turned to her right to open the door to the kitchen, her left foot went over the edge of a landing at the top of the stairs and she stepped into space, falling to the bottom of the stairway, just as Carol's father Hugh had. Nancy survived her fall but suffered serious injuries including a concussion and multiple fractures. I agreed to work for the defense attorney and investigate whether the landing was unsafe and if it complied with the building code or not. After conducting a site inspection and researching codes and standards, I submitted a brief report stating that I was not able to identify any building or housing code violations and the case was settled before the scheduled trial.

It has been interesting for me to think back and compare the similarities and differences between two very similar falls in very similar entryways. One time I was working for the plaintiff, and the other time I was working for the defense.

In both cases the houses, back entrances, landings, and open stairways were very similar. Both falling events were also similar since both Hugh and Nancy were standing on landings at the top of stairways in front of doors when they stepped into space with their left foot. In both cases

I examined the relevant building codes and housing codes but did not identify any violations.

However, there were also some important differences. Where Hugh fell there was a third doorway at the landing, and where Nancy fell there were only two doors at the landing. Another big difference was that the landing where Hugh fell was smaller and there was no room for him to take even one step to his left without stepping into the open stairway. Where Nancy fell, however, the landing was larger, extending 12in. (0.30m) further before the top of the stairway. Another difference was that in Hugh's case there was no lighting issue, but in Nancy's case there was a dispute about whether the lighting was adequate or not at the time of her fall.

If Hugh's case (for the plaintiff) had gone to trial, I would have testified that the landing and stairway were unsafe, and if built today would not comply with the current building code. In Nancy's case the defense attorney who hired me told me he would not be calling on me to testify at trial, and that he just wanted me to research the issues. I reconciled in my mind that I could remain objective in fulfilling my duties as an expert, since my role was to investigate and report what I found and not to take sides.

If the attorneys can work out a settlement, great, but if a case goes to trial, then it is up to the jury to determine who is more negligent, the plaintiff or the defense. However, the burden of proof is always on the plaintiff, and therefore working as an expert for the plaintiff is often more demanding and more time consuming than working for the defense.

A Tub-Shower

Paul Jones and his wife Jane were staying at a downtown hotel. Before dinner Paul decided to take a shower, and while he was in the shower Jane heard a thud, followed by her husband yelling. When Jane entered the bathroom, she realized that Paul had fallen out of the tub-shower and was lying on the floor, lodged against the door. Jane managed to squeeze her way through the door, and after a few minutes Paul said he was ok, just shaken up. Paul told her that he had been washing his foot when he slipped and fell. He said he tried to hold the towel bar on the tub wall, but it broke loose, and he fell outside the tub and onto the floor. That night Paul told Jane he had a migraine headache and went to bed early. He apparently thought it was a migraine since he had a history of them. The next morning when Jane tried to wake up Paul she discovered that he had died during the night. She learned later that Paul's headache was from hemorrhaging or bleeding in the brain.

After much grieving and agony Jane hired an attorney who filed a lawsuit against the hotel. The attorney hired me, and we arranged for a site inspection. On the day of my site inspection the hotel was being extensively remodeled, and the water had been turned off, so I took along a water bottle, a bar of soap, and a small bottle of shampoo. The first thing I realized when I entered the bathroom was how small it was. I understood how Paul hit his head and why Jane had difficulty opening the door after her husband fell. I took measurements and photos of the room and tested the slip resistance at the bottom of the tub. First I took my sock off and stood up in the tub with one bare foot. The surface was dry and was not slippery. Next I wet my foot and the surface of the tub and stood on my foot again. As I moved my foot I detected that the surface was slippery. Next I washed the bottom of my right foot with a small amount of soap and stood up again. This time the surface was very slippery. Finally, I rinsed the soap off my foot and applied a couple of drops of shampoo and some water to my foot and tried to stand again, and this time the surface was extremely slippery.

When Paul fell, the bottom of the tub-shower was both smooth and slippery. The tub did not have a slip resistant finish on the bottom and there was no mat present. The towel bar on the end wall of the tub-shower broke loose when Paul grabbed hold of it. Someone had put it back in place, but it came loose again when I grabbed it. If a securely mounted grab bar had been present instead of a towel bar, he would have had something to grab onto for support.

Towel bars often look similar to grab bars, but towel bars are not designed or manufactured to the same safety specifications as grab bars. Grab bars are required to support a vertical or horizontal force of 250 lbs (1112N). People rely on grab bars to support their weight. Towel bars are intended to hold the weight of towels, maybe five pounds, not the weight of people.

In my report I stated that the owner of the hotel had a responsibility to properly construct and maintain a safe bathroom for public use and that the owner knew, or should have known, that the bottom of the tub was slippery and unsafe without a slip resistant surface or a rubberized mat. I also stated that the owner knew, or should have known, that having a towel bar where there should have been a sturdy grab bar was an unsafe condition, and that people would predictably grab hold of the towel bar for support. The case was settled for a substantial amount before going to trial, and Jane was pleased with the result, although she was still grieving following the death of her husband and would have much preferred it if Paul had never slipped and fallen.

Building codes have continued to improve over the years, but the vast majority of motels, hotels, bed & breakfasts, and AirBnBs, are existing buildings that were constructed when older versions of the building code applied. Another problem is that the lodging industry has not been proactive in fully addressing the issue of slip-resistant surfaces and the installation of grab bars, except where grab bars are required by the ADA Standards. Building codes typically do not require grab bars in all tubs and showers.

When I visit a hotel or motel with no mat or textured surface, I often put a hand towel on the bottom of the tub-shower before I take a shower. I find that I am less likely to slip with a wet hand towel on the bottom of the tub. Fall expert Jake Pauls demonstrated this in a YouTube video he posted. Once you slip and start to fall it is very difficult to stop falling. All of us need to be extremely careful when showering in lodging facilities. Many older buildings have tub-showers that can quickly become slipping hazards, especially when we shampoo or wash our feet. There are often no grab bars, or grab bars are mounted in the wrong places, or there is only one grab bar, or towel bars are placed where there should be grab bars.

Why Did These Falls Result in Death?

The situations described above are a representative sampling of the many investigations I have completed when people died from falls. When I think back to the many investigations I have been involved in over the years, I continue to question why some falls resulted in minor injuries while others resulted in much more serious injuries, and still others resulted in fatalities. For each situation there was a unique set of circumstances, including human behavior and environmental factors, that resulted in a fall. For those unfortunate people who died from their falls, I think back to many "what ifs."

On the human behavior side of the equation, what if Emma Smith had told her daughter that she couldn't manage the high step and had entered the townhouse through the sliding door in back? What if her daughter had asked the building owner to correct the problem? What if Ken Williams had seen the high threshold at the doorway, would he have stepped over it? What if Tyler Walsh had made it a habit to keep a safe distance from the edge of that patio? What if the paramedics had been more cautious when they turned the gurney that Bill Smart was strapped down in? What if Fred Clemens had securely locked the wheels on the wheelchair before his wife Jan sat down in it, would Jan have still fallen and hit her head? What if Sam Sanders had been traveling a bit slower in his electric scooter, would he have still veered off the sidewalk? What if Jim Clover had not taken that last drink before he walked into a dark stairway? What if Hugh Sauer had been consciously aware of how close he was standing to the top of the stairway? What if Paul Jones had not tried to wash the bottom of his feet in the tub-shower?

On the environmental side of things, I wonder what if the step that Emma Smith fell backwards off of had been one inch shorter, would she still have fallen? What if the door threshold where Ken Williams tripped and fell had been painted a bright color or had been one-half inch shorter? What if the grass, that adjoined the patio where Tyler Walsh fell, had been flush and level with the patio, would his walker still have dropped off the edge and would he still have fallen? What if the owner of the nursing home had replaced the broken concrete before the wheels of the gurney got stuck, would Bill Smart still be alive? What if the sidewalk, where Jan Clemens fell while getting into her wheelchair, had better lighting, or if the pavement had been dry, would the wheelchair have slipped, and would she have fallen? What if the cross-slope on the sidewalk where Sam Sanders electric scooter fell off the edge had been two percent instead of almost five percent? What if the stairway where Jim Clover fell had a secure handrail that extended beyond the top of the stairway, would that have made a difference? What if the landing at the top of the stairs where Hugh Sauer fell was one foot wider, would he have still fallen? What if there had been a grab bar in the tub-shower instead of a towel bar, would Paul Jones have slipped and fallen?

We will never know the answers to these questions, yet juries are asked to determine the percentage of responsibility for both the plaintiff and the defense. Almost all of the cases I have investigated over the years, with only a few exceptions, are a complex combination of both human behavior and environmental conditions. Sometimes, but not very often, the individual who dies from a fall has no control over the circumstances of the event, such as when the gurney Bill Smart was in tipped over. So, ask yourself, what do you control in order to reduce your chances of suffering a deadly fall?

Takeaways
Hazards are always all about - but most of them don't stand out
A falling hazard can be present for a long time and can be negotiated by hundreds, or even thousands of people before someone falls. Falls happen suddenly, with almost no time to react. Death can result from tripping at a doorway threshold or falling off a sidewalk or a patio. Individuals can lose their lives from slipping in a shower or falling down a stairway. Most, but not all falls, involve at least some degree

of human error. People should not have to go through life worrying about falling hazards, but unfortunately hazards are so common that people need to maintain a high level of awareness to prevent falls from happening.

Chapter 4

Outdoors: Paths of Unsafe Travel

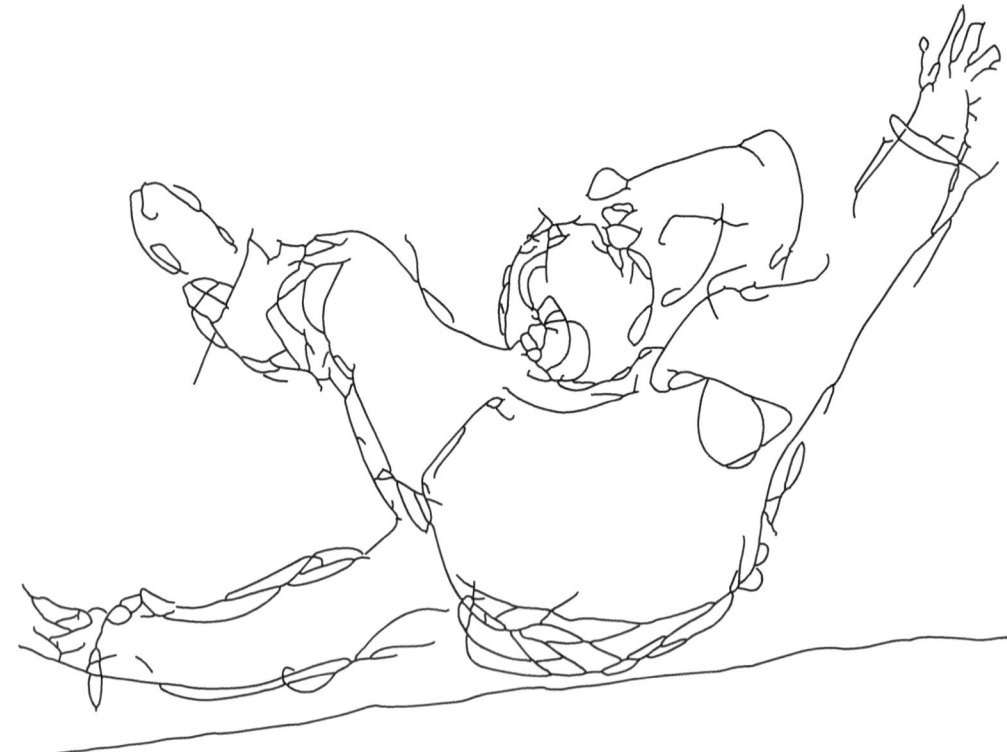

One would think walking on a sidewalk would be a very safe thing to do, and most of the time it is. People get confident on sidewalks and do not think of them as being hazardous. In fact, some people get so confident that they walk backwards while talking to others who are walking behind them. Some people do not pay attention to what they are doing and walk into a street, only to be hit by a 4,000lb (1,814 kg) car traveling at 15mph (24.1km/h)—pretty risky behavior if you ask me. Being overconfident and/or not paying attention can cost you your life.

Sidewalks

Yesterday I was observing my 18-month-old granddaughter walking on a sidewalk, and I noticed that, unlike most adults, she was very cautious and frequently looked down at the surface ahead of her to spot any obstacles that she needed to negotiate. Occasionally she moved too quickly or turned suddenly and ended up falling anyway, but the deliberate moves she made with her eyes and her body were very intriguing to me, and of course when a small child falls from a low height it is usually without serious consequences.

Small elevation changes often occur where 'control joints' are scored every few feet and where 'construction joints' separate different pours of concrete along sidewalks. The changes are subtle and difficult to recognize, but they are also extremely common due to settling and freeze/thaw cycles.

When I was young, it was common knowledge to everyone that stepping on a crack in the walk was 'bad luck'. Now that I am older, I can see the merits of thinking this way, since every crack has the potential of being a tripping hazard. As adults we have become too trusting of the world around us; we assume that we don't have to worry because we have gotten through situations before without problems. But we carry too much, we text and talk while we walk, we neglect to pay enough attention to our surroundings, and we don't look down very often, especially if we have been there before.

We have come to expect walking surfaces that are "flush, stable, and slip resistant," as required by codes and standards. Therefore, when conditions are contrary to what we have come to anticipate, we are more likely to slip, trip, take an airstep, or experience unstable footing. When someone anticipates a wet slippery surface or a tripping hazard ahead, they have a chance to adjust and walk slower and more cautiously. But when someone does not see or anticipate a wet slippery surface or a tripping hazard, the likelihood of a fall increases.

Tripping On Cracks, Hoses, and Curbs

A couple of years ago I tripped and stumbled on a control joint in a sidewalk where a section of concrete had raised up slightly due to frost heave. It happened in the spring while I was walking from my office to teach a class in another building. I had traversed the route a hundred or more times before without incident, but on this particular occasion the toe of my shoe happened to catch on a slight vertical rise at a control joint in the sidewalk. Fortunately, I regained my footing and did not fall to the ground, but because of my interest in falls I decided to go back and examine the deviation that I had failed to observe. I pulled out the small tape measure I carry on my keychain for such occasions, and I discovered that the vertical change in elevation was only 0.25in. (6.4mm). It was difficult to recognize the crack as a tripping hazard, so I was not surprised that I had missed it.

I thought to myself that it was my fault for being careless and not picking up my feet while I was walking, so I went on to teach my class and forgot about it. A couple of days later while passing the same location I saw a student lying on the sidewalk just ahead of where I had tripped. I did not see her fall, but it turned out that she had tripped and fallen in the same location where I had tripped earlier. She hit her face on the pavement and was bleeding but since it did not appear to be serious and other people were attending her, I decided to proceed on to my class.

As the weeks went by, I observed that the height of the vertical change in elevation became more pronounced and the hazard became more visually apparent, and therefore it was more likely to catch my attention so that I consciously stepped over it. The bad thing was that it was now even more of a toe catcher for people who were not paying attention or people who have reduced vision. The university tried patching the joint with a cement patching material. It worked well for a while, but after a couple of months the patching material started to break apart. Eventually a maintenance crew completely removed and replaced the sections of sidewalk on each side of the tripping hazard to reestablish a flush level surface.

Walking is a natural rhythmic cycle that involves constantly shifting your balance and lifting your feet off the walking surface. As you walk, you bounce up and down and swing side to side with each step. It is a highly integrated process that requires ankles, feet, toes, knees and hips to all have a reasonable range of motion, and it helps to have arms that can move freely to maintain balance. Walking is a complex muscular-skeletal and neurological control process. Some researchers have described walking as "controlled falling," or as a continuous series of losses and recoveries of balance, or a series of almost catastrophes.

One might reasonably ask, if there is a change in elevation why don't people see it? For one thing we all tend to look ahead while we are walking, rather than constantly looking down at our feet, which is to be expected. If we spot an elevation change ahead or an obstacle in the route, we tend to make allowances and step over it. But often we do not visually detect the obstacle, or we don't recognize it as a hazard.

Tripping and falling over a small vertical change at a joint in a sidewalk is very common. Your safety depends on your ability to recognize small changes ahead of you. I have lost track of how many lawsuits I have been involved in as expert witness where this was the issue. Sometimes the hazards are hidden or very difficult to visually detect. Other times they are more pronounced and easier to notice.

During normal walking most peoples' toes and heels skim very close to the surface, and it does not take much of a variation in the surface to get caught and stumble. It is difficult to observe this while people are walking, but if you take a slow-motion video of someone walking and play it back, you will understand why this is important. Having adequate toe clearance during the swing phase of your walking cycle will help you avoid tripping, but most of us are not aware of the importance of this until we trip on a deviation in the walking surface. It is well known that a vertical variation in the walking surface of one quarter of an inch or more can be a tripping hazard. Building codes and standards have responded by requiring walking surfaces to be level and flush.

There is also the 'dragging of feet' that many people exhibit. The type and fit of the footwear people have on can also be a factor. Flip-flops and loose sandals are often not as safe as properly fitted shoes. And of course, there is the luck of the circumstances that can occasionally result in the toe of the shoe catching on the vertical hazard.

There are many visual and mental distractions we have to deal with while we walk; looking ahead to see where we are going, watching out for small children, looking at cars, bicyclists, joggers, and dogs. In addition, we have to deal with changing lighting, shadows, glare, and high contrast. There are also sounds that distract us, including the sound of traffic, motorcycles, lawn mowers, trimmers, leaf blowers, and people talking. Things we carry such as small children, pets, grocery bags and purses, and things we push, including strollers and scooters also demand our attention. The side effects of prescription medications, alcohol, and large meals sometimes diminish our alertness, our senses, our response time, and our ability to maintain our center of gravity. For people of advanced age there is also the impact of age-related vision losses, cataracts, muscle stiffness, lack of flexibility, and impaired balance. Glare is a big problem for people with cataracts or other eye diseases. Older adults also need more light to see well than younger people. But despite all of this we keep on walking.

Have you ever been trying to keep up with the person(s) next to you when you found yourself walking faster than the speed you are comfortable with? Walking with someone who walks faster than your normal speed can put you at a greater risk of falling.

When we trip and fall, our first reaction is usually to blame ourselves. "Oh, how careless of me, I should have been walking slower, I should have paid closer attention to what was ahead, I should not have had that beer with my oversized dinner." But when you wake up in the hospital after they removed cartilage to repair your ankle, and the doctor tells you that you will probably have premature arthritis, stiffness, and on and off pain for the rest of your life, you might start to think, "Yes, it was dumb of me, but it was not all my fault, if only that crack in the sidewalk had not been there, I would not be in this situation."

Alicia Herman was walking back to her car after purchasing takeout food at a fast food restaurant when she tripped on a crack in the sidewalk. She fell forward and broke her wrist when she stuck her arm out in front of her in an attempt to break her fall. She broke her fall, but she also broke her wrist.

Alicia's attorney arranged for me to conduct a site inspection. When I arrived at the location, Alicia, her attorney, and the attorney who was representing the restaurant were all present. When I asked Alicia to describe where and how she fell, she pointed out the location and said she did not see the crack before the toe of her shoe caught on the raised edge. Alicia said that it was only after she fell, while she was laying on the sidewalk, that she looked back and realized what she had tripped on.

I inspected the control joint where Alicia tripped. There was a vertical change in elevation that ranged from one half inch at one edge of the sidewalk to 1.5in. (38.1mm) at the other edge of the sidewalk. I noticed that there were additional tripping hazards in other control joints between the restaurant and the parking lot, so I documented those as well.

I observed that the color and texture of the concrete was the same on both sides of the control joint so the surfaces on both sides of the joint blended together visually. This is typical when two sections of concrete are poured on the same day with the same concrete mix. A tripping hazard developed when a full depth crack formed along the control joint, and one section of concrete settled while the other one did not.

In my report I quoted statements from construction industry standards and described the location as non-compliant. I referenced the ADA Standards that require vertical elevation changes in routes to be less than 0.5in. (12.7mm) and to be beveled if between 0.25in. (6.4mm) and 0.5in. (12.7mm). The defense attorney deposed me to record my answers to his questions. During my deposition I provided a detailed description of my research and opinions. The case was settled before going to trial, and Alicia received financial compensation for her injuries.

Places of business, including fast food restaurants, have a responsibility to maintain safe premises. At the restaurant where Alicia fell, the owner had a responsibility to inspect the sidewalk and to identify and correct any hazards. The owner likely knew, or should have known, that a tripping hazard was present and should have provided a warning until the unsafe condition could be corrected. It would have been easy to paint the edges of the tripping hazard on the sidewalk with a bright color to warn people. Unfortunately, tripping hazards like the one Alicia encountered are commonplace.

Molly McQuade parked in front of a gas station/convenience store. The parking spaces in front of the store were taken, so she parked in the end space by the corner of the building. Molly got out of her car, walked to the front of her car, stepped onto the concrete walk, and headed towards the entrance. After taking a couple of steps she tripped over an air hose that was stretched over the sidewalk, she fell and broke her wrist. Molly said in a recorded statement that she was looking ahead to the entrance and did not see the air hose when she tripped over it. Someone had apparently used the air hose but had not wrapped it back up on the hook on the wall. When I inspected the location, the air hose was neatly wrapped up on the hook. However, when Molly fell the air hose draped across the concrete walk in front of the building. Although the air hose was clearly a tripping hazard when Molly fell, I could not identify any codes or standards that applied to the situation. The location of the compressor and air hose created an unsafe condition because when the air hose was not wrapped up on the hook, it became a tripping hazard.

Store owners need to place compressors and air hoses in safe locations away from pedestrian traffic areas because you can't depend on users to always neatly wrap up air hoses. The owner knew that customers often left the air hose draped over the sidewalk and should have moved the compressor and air hose to a safer location. Molly was fortunate to be able to settle the case before trial because a jury might have determined that she was more negligent than the owner of the gas station/convenience store.

Stan White was on his way home from an out-of-town trip when he and his wife Cassy decided to stop at a store to look at some merchandise. They parked in a parking lot in front of the store and walked over to the entrance. Stan was following Cassy as she approached the entrance door. When the toe of his shoe caught on a tapered curb that he did not see, he stumbled forward but was unable to catch himself. Stan fell into the front wall of the building next to the door, hit his head hard against the brick, and broke his neck. Although he experienced limited recovery, Stan will have to live with paralysis for the rest of his life.

I met Stan's attorney at the location where Stan fell. Before taking any photos or measurements I looked over the situation to see if there was anything unusual or out of the ordinary about it. I realized that the curb ramp and sidewalk configuration was not a standard or typical design and then took a series of linear measurements, slope measurements, and photos. I knew that it was a complicated situation that may be difficult to fully explain in my report. I also knew that I would need to research the standards further to determine exactly what complied and what did not, so I made sure I thoroughly documented the existing conditions.

My research revealed that the building originally had a single step up at the entrance door. A contractor was hired to eliminate the step and make the entrance accessible for persons with disabilities. The contractor installed a curb that sloped up from the parking lot to the entrance door. After thoroughly researching the ADA Standards regarding the design of curb ramps, sidewalks, and entrances, I realized that the situation was both unusual and unsafe. As a result, the side-flares (the sloped triangular sections) of the curb ramp were not readily visible because the contactor had blended the concrete surface to connect the curb ramp to an existing sidewalk. In the process of making the curb ramp fit into existing conditions, the contractor had created a non-standard 7.0ft. (2.13m) long tapered curb that sloped from a 4.0in. (101.6mm) curb at one end to a 0.25in. (6.4mm) high tripping hazard at the other end.

The lower portion of the long, tapered curb was very difficult to see because the concrete surfaces of the parking lot, the sidewalk, the curb ramp, and the tapered curb all blended together visually because they had all been installed at the same time. Had the tapered curb been of contrasting color it would have been easier to notice.

In my report to Stan's attorney, I stated my opinion that the owner should have known that the curb ramp and sidewalk configuration did not comply with the ADA Standards and that the long tapered curb was difficult to visually differentiate from adjacent material. I also stated that, since it was in the direct path of travel, the owner of the store should have recognized the tripping hazard and should have painted it a bright color to warn people entering the building until a new curb ramp that was compliant with the ADA Standards could be constructed.

The plaintiff and the defense agreed to mediate the case. The first attempt at mediation—a method of settling a dispute without taking it to trial—failed quickly when it became apparent that the two sides had very different ideas regarding financial compensation. After several depositions—including mine—were taken, the case was mediated again, this time successfully with Stan receiving a large financial settlement. Although Stan and Cassy were pleased with the settlement, they regretted that Stan tripped and fell in the first place because both of them will have to live with the consequences of his injuries for the rest of their lives.

Owners need to know that they may be held accountable for the work their contractors complete when that work does not fully comply with building codes and the ADA Standards. Contractors should not take liberty with the ADA Standards to make things fit because it can lead to unsafe conditions with tragic consequences. Pedestrians need to stay alert for hidden hazards that may be lurking ahead. They should never assume that new construction or modifications are built in full compliance with the ADA Standards, or expect a predictable configuration. When a curb ramp is not a standard design because it was altered to fit existing conditions, it can really throw us off.

Airsteps

Melanie Bartholomew was visiting a friend and was walking on a concrete sidewalk between two apartment buildings when she suddenly fell. She reached out with her hands and arms ahead of her as she fell forward, but she broke her wrist and dislocated her shoulder in the process. Someone nearby heard her yelling and called 911.

The location in the concrete sidewalk where Melanie fell had a single, unmarked step in it. There was grass on both sides of the sidewalk that connected the apartment buildings to the parking lot. I inspected the location, took photos, and measured the height of the step as well as the running and cross-slopes of the sidewalk.

In her deposition Melanie admitted that she had been on the sidewalk before but this time she did not see the single step in front of her before she fell. Melanie said after she fell she looked back and realized that she had missed the step. Since she did not see the step down ahead of her, she continued to walk as if the sidewalk was a level surface and took an 'airstep'. The sections of concrete on both sides of the step in the sidewalk were poured at the same time and were the same color and texture so they blended together, making the step down difficult to recognize.

My report included citations that supported my opinion that the 'one step' situation was unsafe. A single step in a walking path or route is a tripping hazard from one direction and an airstep hazard from the other direction. I noted that there was no warning present and no handrail. At a minimum, the owner could have painted the top and front edges of the step with a bright color to warn pedestrians until the location could be reconstructed to eliminate the single step. I also stated that the single step was in an unexpected location in the middle of a sidewalk, making it very easy to overlook. Melanie was pleased when her attorney was able to settle the case without a trial. A couple of months after the case settled I went back to the location to see if the single step had been eliminated. The step was still there, but at least the top edge and front of the step had been painted with bright yellow paint to warn people.

Unfortunately, single step hazards are far too common. A single step in a path is typically easier to see and recognize as a step up than it is as a step down, but the single step can be hazardous from both directions. Therefore, single steps are unsafe and should be eliminated. Painting the top and front edges with a bright color helps provide warning, but the warning does not correct the unsafe condition. Painting also fades and wears out over time, gets covered with snow, and can be missed by people who are distracted, people who are carrying laundry baskets or other items, and people who have vision loss.

If it is not possible to eliminate a single step in a route, then handrails should be installed on both sides of the step and edge stripping, or permanent marking, should be added to both the top (horizontal) and side (vertical) edges of the step so that it is visible from both directions. However, leaving a single step in a walking path means that the path cannot be, by definition, an 'accessible route.' Most people can't navigate a 7.0in. (0.18m) or 8.0in. (0.2m) step while using a wheelchair, nor should they. If the owner leaves a single step in place, the owner must ensure that there is an alternative accessible path of travel that does not contain a step.

On a clear, sunny day in the spring of the year Melissa McGregor legally parked in a designated accessible parking space in a parking lot in front of a hardware store. When she walked from her car to the entrance, she took an airstep into a pothole that she did not see. She fell and broke her arm.

I met Melissa and her attorney in the parking lot where she fell. The manager and assistant manager of the store and the store's attorney were also present. I immediately observed that the parking lot was in a poor state of repair with many potholes, areas of broken and loose asphalt, and oil stains. After verifying exactly where Melissa fell, I measured the height of the pothole and took slope measurements and photos. The pothole was a depression in the pavement that dropped down more than three inches from the surrounding blacktop. The bottom of the pothole had loose broken asphalt and was partially covered with oil, which made it slippery, increasing the hazard.

In my report I stated that the pothole was a falling hazard in the accessible route from the accessible parking to the building entrance and therefore did not meet the industry standard nor the ADA Standards that requires accessible routes to be "stable, firm, and slip resistant." It also violated the requirement that a vertical change in elevation in the route is not more than 0.5in. (12.7mm). I also stated that the pothole was difficult to see, and the bottom of the pothole was slippery because it was covered with an oily film.

When the hardware store's managers and their attorney watched me taking close up measurements and photos of the parking lot, they likely thought about a jury that would see how bad the deterioration was. They probably also thought about how a jury might sympathize with Melissa's pain and suffering more than sympathizing with the owner of a business who did not maintain the parking lot. Another consideration was that Melissa had a state tag and had legally parked in a designated accessible parking space, and the pothole was in the accessible route from that parking space to the entrance. The attorneys on both sides discussed the matter and the case was settled before going to trial.

Parking lots, especially in northern climates, deteriorate over time and need to be regularly maintained, resurfaced, or replaced. Business owners have an obligation to maintain safe routes from parking areas to entrances, especially for persons with disabilities.

Unstable Footing

Unstable footing often results when we encounter unexpected irregularities in a traveling surface or when there are sloped surfaces, dips or bumps that we don't see. The ADA Standards recognize that cross-slopes (slopes perpendicular to the direction of travel) in excess of 2% (or just 0.75in. (19.1mm) change drop in a 3ft. (0.91m) wide walk) can be hazardous, but unfortunately cross-slopes of four to six percent or more are common. That is enough to throw off someone's footing and balance, especially if you don't recognize the slope.

Side flares at curb ramps are typically triangular shaped sections of concrete that slope in two directions. The ADA Standards have maximum slope requirements for side flares, but poor design, poor quality control during construction, and the practice of making side flares steeper to fit into existing sidewalks often results in severe and hazardous slopes.

Terry Cutler fell and broke his foot and ankle as a result of unstable footing when he stepped off of the end of a concrete walk in front of an equipment supply store. After shopping, he walked down the sidewalk and fell while stepping onto the gravel parking lot at the end of the sidewalk.

A suit was filed against the store owner and Terry's attorney hired me to assess the conditions. When I arrived at the site I measured the running-slope (the slope in the direction of travel) of the sidewalk where Terry fell, and determined it was 13.5% which is significantly more than the ADA Standard maximum slope for an accessible route or a ramp. Since the store was constructed well after the ADA became law, the business was required to have designated accessible parking spaces, an accessible route to the entrance, and a grade level accessible entrance.

The business did have accessible parking spaces and an accessible entrance, but the route in between was too steep. Since it did not meet the slope requirement for a route, it should have been designed as a ramp and should have met all of the requirements for ramps including maximum slope, landings, handrails, and handrail extensions. However, the sidewalk was very steep and there was no landing at the end of the sidewalk where Terry fell. There were also no handrail extensions for him to grab onto when he stepped off the steep concrete walk and onto the parking lot. Another problem was that the gravel at the end of the concrete walk was 2.0in. (50.8mm) lower, so when Terry stepped off the sloped walk and onto the gravel parking lot he experienced unstable footing, twisted his ankle and fell. He stated in his deposition that, after he fell, he tried to stand up, but soon realized he couldn't because he had no control of his right leg which was in severe pain. Terry had two surgeries on his ankle and did not fully recover the feeling in his toes due to nerve and bone damage.

In my deposition I testified that the location where Terry fell did not comply with the ADA Standards because the sidewalk was too steep and it should have been designed as a ramp with handrail extensions and a flat level landing at the bottom, without a 2.0in. (50.8mm) drop. Terry was pleased that the case was settled without having to go to trial.

Barbara Jenkins fell as a result of unstable footing following an outdoor concert as she walked back to a parking lot. Barbara was recovering from a broken leg and was using crutches when she fell, so the uneven and unpaved path she was using was especially treacherous for her. As she walked along the path her right crutch slipped out from the uneven surface and she lost her footing and started to fall. There was nothing to prevent her from falling 5.0 ft. (1.5m) to a terrace below and she landed directly on top of Arnold, who was laying on the ground waiting for the crowd to thin out. Without warning or time to react and get out of the way, Arnold was hit by Barbara's flying body. Arnold was severely injured, but Barbara was fortunate not to be injured at all.

I was hired by Arnold's attorney. During my site inspection I identified three unsafe conditions on the path; excessive cross-slope, uneven surfaces, and no guardrails along the open side of the path to protect someone from falling to the terrace below.

I determined that the ADA Standards were not applicable because the path was not intended or required to be an accessible route. There were also no code violations that were applicable. However, I did conclude that the path was unsafe and that, given the frequency of heavy usage following concerts, the owner should have maintained safe paths of travel to the parking lot. In my report I referred to design and construction standards for routes of travel, and I stated that the owner had a responsibility to ensure that the path was free of hazards.

The case was settled to Arnold's satisfaction before going to trial. While it is rare to have someone suddenly fall on top of you, this is an example of how anybody can become a victim of a falling incident.

Slipping

Kimberly Parker was taking her children trick-or-treating when she slipped and fell on her neighbor's mud-covered sidewalk. It was dark, so Kimberly was using her smart phone as a flashlight while she followed her children who had walked ahead of her. When she stepped on the mud covered section of the sidewalk her right foot slipped out in front of her and she lost her balance. Unfortunately her left foot stayed back and that resulted in a fractured leg. Her daughter heard her yelling and immediately went back to assist her, but the damage had already been done. A neighbor came over to watch the children while Kimberly was taken to the hospital.

The attorney sent me photos and Kimberly's deposition to review. Kimberly said in her deposition that she was aware of the mud and was using caution while walking on the sidewalk, but she slipped and fell anyway. Evidence in the case showed that the sidewalk was in a poor state of repair with multiple cracks and broken surfaces. The homeowner had been notified earlier by the city that it was the duty of the property owner to make improvements to the sidewalk. The city code of ordinances also required property owners to keep sidewalks clean of accumulations of mud, sand, and other debris.

The homeowner had been remodeling and making grading changes around the perimeter of the house but had not yet corrected all the drainage problems. When it rained, water soaked into the exposed soil and a muddy mix spilled over the sidewalk.

I submitted a report articulating the unsafe conditions and the homeowner's obligation to barricade the unsafe section of sidewalk until the problems could be corrected, and fortunately for Kimberly the case was settled without having a trial.

Slipping on muddy sidewalks can be problematic for people that are walking, but it can also be a problem for people using bicycles, electric scooters, and other devices. On a bright sunny day recently I was riding my Segway when I encountered a patch of mud covering the sidewalk. As I approached it I thought I would just proceed slowly, but suddenly the two rubber-tire wheels went out from under me and I fell and hit hard on the concrete. Fortunately I was able to land on my side and roll out the fall, but I still experienced a scraped elbow and multiple aches and pains. The Segway spun out of control and landed 12.0ft (3.7m) in front of me on its side as it automatically shut off. I laid on the ground for a minute or two to make sure nothing was broken. I was wearing a helmet, a long sleeve shirt, and long pants which fortunately helped prevent more serious injury.

It seems that some lessons are best learned from direct experience, and this was one of them for me. I had no idea I was at risk of slipping and falling, and I was fortunate not to get seriously hurt, but from this day forward I will avoid traveling over muddy sections of sidewalk, or get off my Segway, turn it off and walk it over the grass to the dry sidewalk ahead.

Karen Nelson slipped and fell when she took a shortcut up a grassy hillside to watch her niece play softball. When Karen arrived at the site, the parking lots were full, so she parked in a grassy area off to the side of the road. Since there was no direct route available from where she parked to the softball field, she decided to walk around the end of a fence and up a hillside where she slipped on damp grass, fell and broke her ankle and her wrist.

Karen's attorney hired an expert who contended that the site was unsafe, and the owner should have extended the fence to prevent people from taking a shortcut. The expert stated in his report that the owner should have known that people would take a shortcut up the hill. He also made a general statement that the location did not comply with codes and standards but did not cite any specific codes or code violations.

In my report for the defense I stated that there were no code violations and that Karen was aware of the fact that there was a safe concrete walk to the softball field, but she chose to take a hazardous shortcut up the hillside rather than a longer and safer route.

The softball field's owner did not offer to settle, and consequently the case went to trial. The jury found for the defense and no financial compensation was awarded to Karen. During the trial the plaintiff's attorney failed to specify any violations of codes or standards and also failed to convince the jury that the owner should have continued the fence to prevent people from walking up the hillside.

This should be a lesson to all of us. Take shortcuts at your own risk. Damp grass on a hillside can be slippery, so if you want to play it safe, take the longer way around. And if you do take a shortcut and fall and get injured, don't assume that a jury will side with you. Jurors are typically sympathetic to the pain and suffering that results from falls, but that does not mean that they will find the owner to be more negligent than you were.

You can reduce your chances of falling outside by sharpening your observation skills, improving your ability to negotiate hazards, and learning how to fall without getting injured.

Walking Safely On Exterior Routes
Assume paths are unsafe
- Stay aware of your surroundings and watch out for falling hazards
- Look carefully when lighting conditions or shadows obscure your vision

Don't get tripped up
- Watch out for trippers (height differences and/or gaps between sections of sidewalks that can catch the toe of your shoe)
- Remember that as little as 0.25in. (6.4mm) can trip you up
- Be on the lookout for material changes ahead of you (concrete to asphalt, brick to concrete, etc.)
- Look for slightly raised sections of concrete near manhole covers, drainage areas, and trees
- Watch for raised metal grate edges that surround trees in sidewalks
- Walk cautiously on irregular stone or brick surfaces
- Watch out for tapered curbs near curb ramps and building entrances
- Be aware of wheel stops that may be tripping hazards

Don't get slipped up
- Wear properly fitting, slip-resistant footwear
- Be aware of your body position and your footing when getting

in and out of vehicles, especially when parking areas are snow covered, wet, or icy

Take it slow on ice and snow
- Walk slower and allow extra time when wet or slippery conditions exist
- Walk at your own comfortable pace and don't try to keep up with others in slippery conditions
- If you suspect a slippery area ahead, tap your foot on it while hanging on to something solid if you can before walking on it
- If you walk on slippery surfaces, take short steps and walk 'flat-footed', keeping your center of gravity over your support leg as much as possible
- Try to avoid carrying items, or use a backpack to keep your arms free to move for balancing
- Watch out for black ice (a thin layer of ice that is difficult to see) on paved surfaces especially on dark asphalt
- Watch out for loose material including mulch, gravel, twigs, leaves, paper, trash, and small rocks on sidewalks
- Consider walking on the grass next to the sidewalk if the sidewalk is more slippery than the grass

Don't allow unstable footing or airsteps to throw you down
- Watch out for sloped surfaces in various directions, especially at curb ramps and driveways
- Learn to observe excessive cross-slopes ahead that might twist your ankle or throw off your balance
- Watch out for airstep hazards in sidewalks, at the sides and ends of sidewalks, at doorways, and at depressions in parking lots
- Watch out for lower surfaces along the edges and at the ends of sidewalks that may result in a miss-step

Takeaways
I was walking too fast - now the pain and strain will last

For most of us walking is second nature and we do not think about every step we take. Walking on two feet involves constantly shifting our center of gravity, and since falling hazards are commonplace and often difficult to recognize, it does not take much to throw off our balance. A small crack in the sidewalk is all it takes to trip someone up and stepping onto a slippery surface can cause someone's feet to suddenly fly out from under them. Single steps frequently go unnoticed and often lead to missteps and falls. When single steps are in unexpected locations they are especially hazardous.

Chapter 5
Entrances: Proceed at Your Own Risk

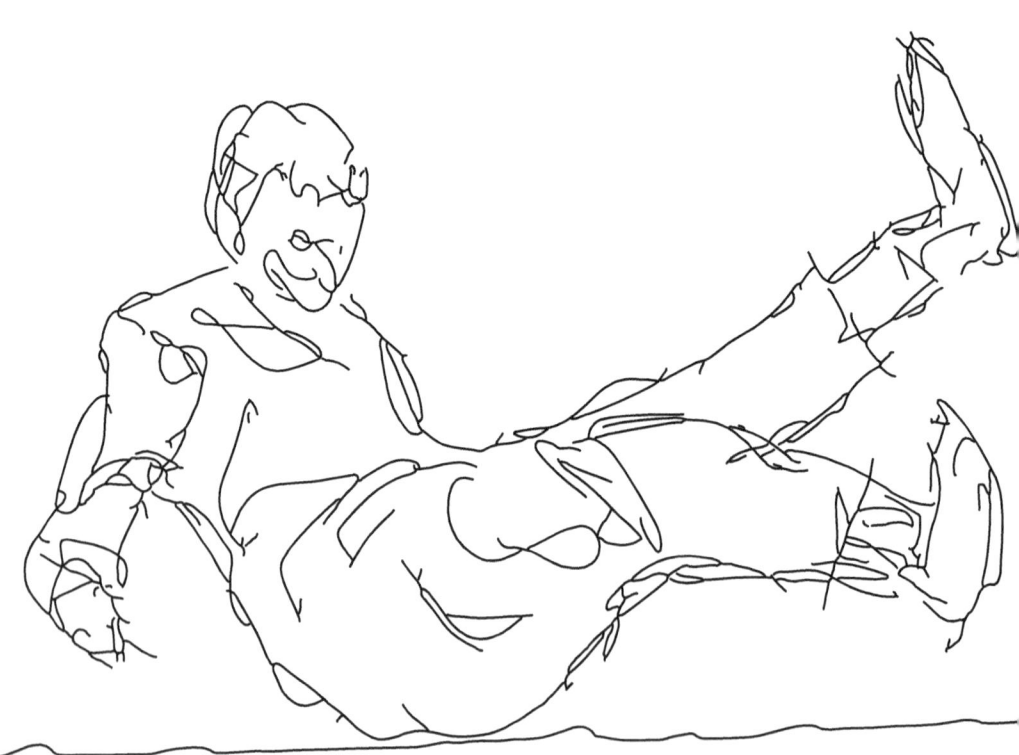

Why Are Falls At Doorways So Common?

We are often distracted as we walk in and out of buildings, and unfortunately falls occur frequently at entrances and doors. Sometimes we are looking at and/or speaking to others, holding doors open for others, or thinking about where we parked. Entering unfamiliar interiors with changing lighting levels requires our adjustment, and when our mobile phones ring, the last thing on our minds is to consciously think about where we are walking.

Tripping at doorways is common because so many doorways have high instead of low-profile thresholds (the transition at the bottom of the doorway). When there is a high threshold or a single step present at a doorway, we are more likely to fall. If we shuffle our feet or use a mobility device such as a cane, wheelchair, or walker, high thresholds at doors are especially problematic. Airsteps happen at doorways when people walking through them unexpectedly experience a drop of as little as one inch. Often it is difficult to recognize these changes because surfaces of the same color or material appear to blend together and look like one flat continuous surface.

After someone falls, owners of buildings that are open to the public often paint the edges of high thresholds and single steps at doorways a bright color to provide a warning, but a warning does not correct an unsafe condition. Therefore owners should think of warnings as temporary measures until the unsafe conditions can be corrected. I believe all high thresholds and single steps at doorways into public buildings, even small ones, should be eliminated.

Small businesses in downtown areas are particularly problematic because many of them have excessively sloped sidewalks leading up to entrances where steps have been removed. This is ironic because steps at entrances were eliminated to provide wheelchair access, but if it was not done correctly it creates another hazard, namely excessive slopes. Sometimes the doors themselves can be hazardous when they are too large or heavy, or when they have poor quality closing devices. Open sides of raised landings (flat-level platforms) at doorways are another common falling hazard when they are either too small and/or not equipped with handrails or guardrails.

Entrances and Doorways

Mary Jones tripped, fell, and broke her wrist while walking through the entrance door at a restaurant. When I inspected the doorway I determined that the location where Mary fell was unsafe because the metal threshold at the bottom of the doorway had a 2.0 in. (50.8mm) high gap underneath it. The gap extended back underneath the metal edge by more than 1.0in. (25.4mm), making it a perfect toe-catching cavity. Although hundreds of people had successfully navigated the doorway before Mary without incident, it was a tripping hazard waiting for someone to find it.

Mary said in her deposition that she put her right foot on the floor inside the doorway but when she tried to move her left foot up, it caught in the gap, and she fell onto her side and could not move. She fell on her hip and broke her pelvis in five places. Previous to her fall she had been diagnosed earlier as having osteoporosis, which helps explain the severity of her injuries. Mary said in her deposition that she will never fully recover, and she moves slower now, and it takes her more time to get things done.

In my report I said that the only viable mitigation to make the location safe and in compliance with the building code and the ADA Standards was to remove the concrete landing outside the door and replace it with new concrete to match up with the inside floor level. This would eliminate the toe catcher beneath the metal threshold and make the landing outside the door flush with the bottom of the threshold. I stated that it would be appropriate to maintain a modest 2% slope away from the doorway for drainage, but the cavity under the threshold should be eliminated.

Mary was pleased that her attorney was able to settle the case before the scheduled trial date, but she also realized that she would have to live with the consequences of her fall for the rest of her life.

Mandy Ramirez fell as she walked out of a restaurant to go back to her parked car. She had used the front door when she entered the restaurant but walked out the side door when she left because it was closer to her car. Since she had never exited through the side door before, she did not realize that there was a step down to a concrete sidewalk. Mandy took an airstep, fell forward, suffered a concussion, and broke her jaw and cheekbone.

It was a bright summer day outside when she fell, and Mandy had been inside the dimly lit interior of the restaurant for an hour before leaving, so when she stepped outside, her eyes did not have time to adjust to the bright sunlight. She said in her deposition that when she walked out the doorway she was momentarily blinded by the bright light. When I measured the lighting level on the floor inside the door it was less than 0.1 foot-candle (one tenth of one foot candle or 1.09 lumens), which is well below the minimum standard for safety set by the Illuminating Engineering Society of North America. Lighting outside on a bright sunny day can be as much as 10,000 foot-candles (107,527 lumens), so it is not surprising that she did not notice the step down.

After checking applicable codes and standards, I concluded that the presence of the single step at the required exit doorway was a violation of the International Building Code, the Life Safety Code, and the ADA Standards. The Life Safety Code requires that occupants of a building must be protected from obstacles to safely egress. Single steps at doorways are hazardous because they frequently go unnoticed and, as a consequence, result in tripping going in and airsteps going out. Additionally, there was no sign posted to "Watch your step." Although there was no requirement in the building code or the life safety code to post a warning, Mandy probably would not have fallen if there had been a prominently placed warning at the door. I was able to write a comprehensive report and cite specific code violations and Mandy received a settlement before the case was scheduled for trial.

Portable Ramps and Landings

Steve and Brenda Dutton went to lunch at a local restaurant in the small town near where they lived. After lunch they left through the same doorway in the back of the restaurant where they had parked. However, when they walked through the doorway this time there was a portable ramp sitting over the 2.0 in. (50.8mm) high threshold. It had been placed there earlier so another customer using a wheelchair could enter. Brenda was walking ahead of Steve when she heard Steve fall off the ramp behind her. She turned around and went back to find Steve lying motionless on the pavement at the bottom of the ramp. Brenda went back into the doorway and called out for help, then she walked down the ramp again to attend to her husband. Then Brenda also fell off the ramp and although her injuries were minor, Steve's were serious. He was rushed to the hospital and admitted to an intensive care unit, but Steve died three weeks later from the injuries he suffered in the fall.

Following my review of documents and photos, I concluded that the portable ramp should not have been left in place at the doorway because it created an unsafe condition. The high threshold was a hazard, but the portable ramp that was left in place over the threshold was even more hazardous.

The three-foot-long portable folding ramp had aluminum plates hinged at both ends. The plates at one end laid on the concrete parking lot and the plates at the other end laid over the threshold, but were not flat on the floor. Instead they angled up to the end of the ramp and then angled down towards the parking lot. Steve may have lost his footing as he stepped onto the sloped plates, or as he stepped onto the ramp itself, or he may have fallen off the side of the ramp. He may also have caught his toe in the gap between the aluminum plate and the floor. Regardless of what caused him to fall, walking on the portable ramp was hazardous. Since no one actually saw Steve fall, we will never know exactly what caused him to lose his balance. I submitted my report describing the unsafe conditions and the case was settled for a substantial amount before the scheduled trial date.

Portable ramps have their place, but their use should be carefully supervised, and they should not be left in locations like entrance doorways at restaurants where people have no choice but to walk over them to enter and exit.

Susan Greenleaf was sitting at the top of the stairs in front of her apartment building, drinking a cup of coffee. When another resident came up the stairs carrying a baby in one arm and a bag of groceries in the other, Susan got up and opened the door for her. While holding the cup of coffee in her left hand she opened a door at the top of the stairs with her right hand. When she stepped back on the landing to hold the door open and make room for the resident to enter, Susan stepped back and fell off the landing. There was no handrail or guardrail present to prevent her from stepping backwards off the edge, and she fell onto the ground and severely twisted and injured her leg and knee when she hit the ground. Susan had walked in and out of the front door many times before without incident, but this time when she held the door open, she did not realize how close she was to the edge of the landing.

The building was constructed in the 1960s with a stairway consisting of seven risers leading up to a landing at the front door. There was no handrail present on the right side of the stairs, and there was no guardrail on the side of the landing. The building code requires a guardrail on the open sides of landings where the height of the landing is thirty inches or greater. Since the height of the landing was over thirty inches it should have been equipped with a guardrail. However, with no handrail or guardrail present, there was nothing to prevent Susan from falling backwards off the landing.

It was evident from photos that a handrail had once been present, but rusty holes in the concrete were all that remained where metal posts had once been attached. In my report I stated my opinion that not replacing the missing railing clearly showed negligence on the part of the building owner, and even though the stairway and landing may have complied with the building code when it was constructed, the building was not maintained to comply with the building code since the missing handrail had not been replaced.

The defendants filed a 'motion for summary judgment' to have the case dismissed by the court before trial. The defense argued that since Susan had lived in the building for five years, she should have been familiar with the stairway and landing. The defense also argued that the 'negligence per se' argument was not applicable because there was no evidence of a building code violation. They also argued that the apartment building owner did not know that there were any code violations.

The court denied the defendant's motion and settlement discussions led to an agreement that was acceptable to Susan, so a trial was avoided.

Sliding Doors

Tyson Purdy was a frail gentleman in his 80s. He was leaving a discount store when a sliding power door closed suddenly, hit him hard, and knocked him over. He suffered a broken hip and died later from complications. Tyson's daughter Christina was with him when he fell. However, she had walked out of the store a few steps ahead of Tyson. When she heard him cry out, Christina turned around and saw her father lying on the floor.

The defense did not accept Christina's story that the door had knocked Tyson over because she did not actually witness his fall. The defense also contended that "a power door does not just hit someone and knock them over."

When I met Christina's attorney on site, I walked through the automatic sliding doorway several times to determine if it was working properly. When it became apparent that it was not working smoothly or consistently, I got out my video camera and asked the attorney I was working for to stand behind me and take a video while I walked slowly through the doorway, as Tyson had. The door opened properly, but when I walked slowly through the open doorway, the door suddenly closed on me, clobbering my left side and shoulder. I did not fall over, and I was not hurt (and no, I did not file my own lawsuit). However, I certainly understood how Tyson, who was frail and had difficulty walking, could have been easily knocked over.

The attorney representing the store was present during my site inspection and watched as the door hit me. He also saw us taking the video. Common sense would lead one to believe it would be very unlikely that a person would get hit by, let alone be knocked over by a sliding door, but in this case there was enough force to do exactly that. In hindsight, it is unfortunate that Christina did not hold her father's arm and escort him through the doorway. However, it is totally understandable that she did not, because one does not expect an automatic door to malfunction and hit a person.

My report detailed why the automatic door system was unsafe. It was an older system with obsolete technology that did not have redundant high and low infrared sensors at the doorway. Redundant systems increase safety and have become the accepted industry standard. The system was also poorly maintained and was not working properly when the door knocked Tyson over. The store settled with Christina who received an undisclosed amount.

Takeaways

I was on my own - looking at my phone - when I suddenly fell and started to moan

Single steps at doorways and doorways with high thresholds are common trip and airstep hazards. Changes in light levels and distractions can increase the danger at doorways. Inadequately sized landings at the top of stairs or outside doorways, or landings that do not have proper handrails or guardrails, can also be falling hazards. And although it is not likely that an automatic door will knock a person over, it does happen.

Chapter 6
Indoors: Step Carefully

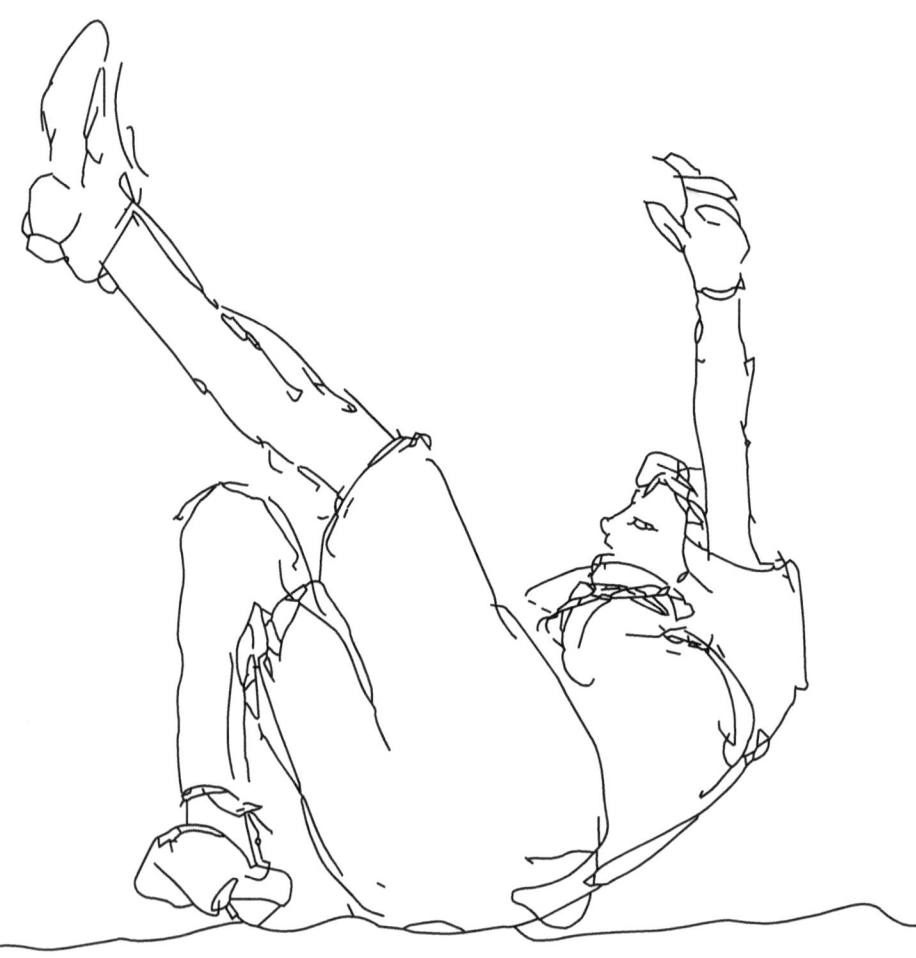

Flooring Materials

You might assume that you are less likely to slip and fall indoors than you are outdoors. However, the Consumer Product Safety Commission (CPSC) estimates that floors and flooring materials directly contribute to more than two million fall injuries annually (National Floor Safety Institute [NFSI] website). Although the ADA Standards for accessible routes are the same for both exterior and interior routes, falling hazards indoors are often more difficult to observe than they are on exterior surfaces. Slip-and-fall expert Russell Kendzior authored a book on the subject entitled Falls Aren't Funny that includes discussions about slipping hazards on different types of flooring surfaces and materials, appropriate and inappropriate cleaning/polishing products and procedures, and floor materials and footwear. The interior falls that were caused by slips that I have investigated have typically involved smooth flooring materials that became slippery when wet.

Slipping on Floors

Mindy Halverson slipped, fell and broke her wrist on a wet floor as she walked towards the exit in a grocery store. After making a purchase Mindy walked through a check-out lane and while she was walking past the other check-out lanes her feet suddenly went out from under her. The store's surveillance video clearly showed her slipping and falling.

A sales associate attempted to clean up the spill before Mindy fell, but liquid from the spill had seeped out onto the floor beyond the end of the checkout lane.

The defense argued that there was a wet floor warning sign and a mop and bucket in the area and that Mindy should have seen them and proceeded with caution. After reviewing the surveillance video a few more times, and after reading Mindy's recorded statement, it was evident that those items were located in the checkout lane, but Mindy did not see them because she slipped and fell beyond the end of the checkout lane, where the liquid had spread. Mindy's account of what happened was credible and the defense realized it would have a difficult time overcoming a jury's reaction to the surveillance video, so they wisely settled the case before trial.

Amanda Womack slipped, fell, and broke her wrist while she was working her shift at a big-box store in the early morning before the store opened. She slipped and lost her balance while walking down a corridor to take a break in the employee lounge. Fortunately for Amanda, there was a surveillance video that showed her slipping and falling. When I reviewed the video, it was evident that she was not aware that the vinyl floor was wet. She was walking in a normal manner when she slipped, and her feet suddenly went out from under her. Another surveillance video taken a few minutes earlier of the same location showed a man riding a large floor cleaning and polishing machine before Amanda fell. Following my review of both videos I had a conference call with Amanda and her attorney. She confirmed that she did not know that the floor was wet until she was lying on the floor and realized her clothes and hands were wet, and her wrist hurt. Amanda's account of what happened was very consistent with what I saw on the surveillance video. I submitted a report, and the case settled before going to trial.

Tripping Indoors

Mike Andrews was walking in a store when he tripped and fell. He broke his arm and dislocated his shoulder. Mike's attorney asked me to assess the conditions where Mike fell. The floor was a continuous, level concrete surface, but when carpeting was installed over a portion of the floor a transition strip was added along the edge of the carpeting that had a 0.38in. (9.0mm) high vertical edge. A vertical elevation change along an accessible route that is more than one quarter inch (but less than the 0.5in. or 12.7mm) is permitted by the ADA Standards but only if it has a tapered edge. In this case the elevation change exceeded 0.25in. (6.4mm) and was vertical, so it did not comply with the standards. I know from my own experience that it is easy to catch the toe of my shoe on a small vertical change in elevation.

In my report I stated that the transition strip was a tripping hazard that did not comply with the ADA Standards. Fortunately for Mike the case was settled before trial, and he received adequate financial compensation.

Julie Jones was shopping at a big-box store and was on her way to the restroom when the toe of her shoe caught on a transition from a concrete floor to a tile floor at a restroom doorway. Julie fell and broke her elbow and decided to file a lawsuit. Julie's attorney contacted me, and we arranged a time to conduct a site inspection. When we met at the store, I realized that when tile was installed over a concrete floor in the restroom, the contractor neglected to install a sloping transition strip at the doorway. The result was a vertical change in level at the edge of the doorway that was 0.5in. (12.7mm).

Since the elevation change exceeded 0.25in. (6.4mm), and there was no tapered edge, it did not comply with the ADA Standards. I stated in my report that the ADA Standards were developed to ensure that environments are safe and accessible for all people, and not just wheelchair users. The case was settled, and Julie received adequate financial compensation without having to go through a trial.

These types of tripping hazards are unfortunately very commonplace, and all of us need to constantly watch our step, especially when walking over transitions between flooring materials. Building owners and carpet and tile installers need to ensure that flooring material changes are not tripping hazards. Sloped, low-profile, securely attached transition strips are needed.

A classic tripping hazard is the entry floor mat. Heather Duke found the rolled-up edge of a floor mat with her foot while entering the lobby of a bank. She fell forward, sprained her wrist and broke her arm. Fortunately, I was able to conduct my site inspection for the defense one week after Heather fell. This is unusual because I am often asked to conduct a site inspection after months have passed and improvements have been made. I was able to verify that nothing had been changed in the lobby between the time Heather fell and the day I conducted my site inspection. The floor mats at the bank were provided by an outside vendor who changed them out and cleaned them on a regular basis, but I was able to confirm that the floor mat I inspected was indeed the same floor mat that Heather tripped on.

It is easy to catch the toe of your shoe on the loose edge of a floor mat, so my first thought was, "did they really need to hire an expert for this?" I knew when I was contacted by the defense attorney that I would not need to spend much time on the case, but at his request I agreed to conduct a site inspection and provide my opinion. My inspection of the floor mat revealed that there was nothing unusual about it. It was a high-quality mat with a substantial, rubberized edge that gripped to the tile floor underneath it.

I spoke with the attorney after my inspection and told her all floor mats are a potential tripping hazard, but some styles and types are more hazardous than others. Those that have outer edges that flip up and catch toes are particularly bad, while other heavy mats with heavy tapered edges tend to stay in place, unless they have excessive wear. I reported that I did not know of any building codes or industry standards that were not adhered to. The defense offered a low settlement amount and Heather accepted the offer.

Both parties acted responsibly in reaching an agreement. If the matter had gone to trial, the plaintiff may have had a difficult time obtaining the sympathy of the jury. If the floor mat had been old and worn out with a poor grip and loose edges, the plaintiff would have had a stronger argument.

In another case Carl Noble fell and broke his arm while entering a newly constructed office building when the toe of his shoe caught on the leading edge of a floor mat. According to his account of the event, he tripped on the gathered end of a mat. He said the end of the mat flipped up as he fell forward onto the floor and then flopped back down, flat on the floor.

In my report I stated my opinion that the floor mat was unsafe because it was a thin, worn out mat of poor quality that was not securely attached to the floor and that the owner had a responsibility to remove or replace the unsafe floor mat. I also stated that a better alternative to a loose floor mat would be an integrated floor mat system where the floor mat is recessed so that the edges of the mat are flush with the surrounding floor. Integrated floor mat systems are commonly used in new commercial and institutional buildings. If there had been an integrated floor mat that was properly secured and flush with the floor, Carl would not have tripped and fallen. The case settled before the scheduled trial date.

In much of the country large floor mats are commonplace inside entrances. They are typically used to catch snow, sand, and salt deposits from boots and shoes, and to minimize moisture and debris being carried into the building. Worn out or flimsy floor mats are common tripping hazards, so mats should be cleaned often, inspected often, and replaced or eliminated when they begin to slip, curl, or wrinkle.

Unstable Footing and Airsteps

On a bright, sunny afternoon Tina Buckley decided to go to a movie at a local theatre. When Tina walked into the dark theatre, commercials were being shown on the screen. She was wearing leather sandals and carrying a purse as she walked down a cross aisle that paralleled the movie screen. When she looked to her left to scan for empty seats she stumbled and fell on what her attorney referred to as "a wheelchair ramp." She stuck both hands out to try and break her fall but then severely injured both of her shoulders when she hit the floor hard.

I met Tina, her attorney, and the defense attorney at the movie theatre. We arrived in the morning before the first movie showing. Tina identified the location where she fell and explained the circumstances of her fall. The theatre had installed plastic tubes with small LED lights along the edges of the aisles to help a person see the edges, but the lighting on the floor surface itself was very low when the house lights were dimmed. I took measurements, slope measurements, light readings and photos of the location. Then the assistant manager of the theatre explained how the computerized lighting sequence in the theatre worked. Then he started the sequence, and I took a series of light readings at the floor surface and at waist level on the sloped floor where Tina fell. The computerized lighting sequence had four lighting levels: 1) the brightest level with all of the house lights on full (while staff clean up the floors between shows); 2) the second lighting level with the house lights off and theatre lights partially dimmed (during commercials); 3) the third lighting level with theatre lights dimmed further (during previews); and 4) the fourth lighting level with theatre lights dimmed to their lowest level (during the showing of the movie). My lighting measurements determined that during commercials, previews, and the movie, the light readings on the sloped floor where Tina fell were all below the minimum levels established by the Illuminating Engineering Society of North America (IES).

The carpet that covered both the aisle floor and the sloped floor was a dark color, and although the slope of the floor was not excessive, it was very difficult to recognize that the floor was sloped at all. I could see how it could throw off Tina's footing and balance when she stepped on it.

In my report I stated that the location was unsafe when Tina fell due to the combination of several conditions; 1) a sudden change from a flat aisle floor to a sloped aisle floor, 2) the presence of dark carpeting that continued over both the flat and sloped floor, and 3) the extremely low lighting level. I also stated that it would have been easy for the owner of the theatre to improve the safety of the location by increasing the lighting on the sloped floor surface and by changing the carpet color on the sloped surface to provide better contrast. These interventions would have been easy and inexpensive to accomplish and would likely have prevented the fall.

At trial the jury determined that the theatre was more negligent than Tina was, and Tina was awarded a significant amount for damages. The jury agreed with the plaintiff's contention that the location was a hidden and unmarked hazard that anyone could have fallen on. The jury also believed that the owner should have recognized the problem and corrected it.

Raised restaurant booths are not welcoming and unsafe for a major segment of the population. I have been contacted several times by attorneys concerning situations where people stumbled and fell after eating at their booths where the booths were six to eight inches above the floor level. However, only one of the fall cases was pursued after I reported to the attorneys that raised booths were common, and that I was not aware of any codes or standards that prohibit raised booths. However, when raised booths are provided, the ADA Standards require at least five percent of those booths (or at least a minimum of one) to be accessible for people using wheelchairs and for people that have difficulty negotiating steps.

In one of the falls I was contacted about, Donna Sharpe stood up in the booth to visit the restroom but momentarily forgot she was above the main floor level when she miss-stepped and fell. Donna essentially stepped into space instead of stepping onto the floor. The floor in the booth was covered with a textured multicolored carpeting, but the same carpeting was present in the booth and on the floor next to the booth, so all the surfaces visually blended together, making the step very difficult to see. Additionally, the edge of the step was not marked to add visual contrast, and there were no railings or hand holds present on the sides of the booth. The step was also at the edge of the booth, making it more difficult to recognize the change in elevation since there was no platform to stand on before stepping down to the main floor. Although I was not able to identify any building code violations, the attorney asked me to write a report describing the unsafe condition. Fortunately for Donna the attorney was able to settle the case.

The best practice would be to not have raised booths or steps at the edges of booths at all. However, when steps are present at booths, several design interventions should be implemented to improve safety. The overall lighting level at the floor surface and at the edge of the steps should be increased. The floor surfaces of the booth should be of contrasting color to the floor surface of the floor below, or alternatively, a bright colored strip should be installed at the step edge to make the transition more easily recognizable. Additionally, vertical grab bars should be mounted on the vertical wing walls between the booths. Grab bars act as visual cues to alert people that a step is present. They also provide something for people to hold onto as they step in and out of raised booths.

My advice to users is: always be cautious and aware of your surroundings, don't sit in raised booths if your little voice tells you not to, and don't sit in raised booths if you, or someone you are with, has poor vision and/or memory problems. My advice to restaurant and bar owners is, don't build raised booths in the first place, but if you have them, take appropriate measures to make them safer, and make sure you have good legal representation.

Several of my investigations have involved airstep falls indoors. People have walked off podiums, platforms, stages, and single steps. To visualize how fast an airstep can happen, watch the famous video clip of a fall by Fidel Castro in 2004. After one of his long speeches, he walked straight ahead and missed a step that he obviously did not see. He turned and avoided hitting his head, but he suffered a broken shoulder and a broken knee cap. When you watch the video clip you realize how quickly an airstep can occur and how serious it can be.

Takeaways
I slipped - I tripped - I stumbled - I fell

There are many ways to fall indoors in public buildings. Once inside, people can slip on wet or highly-polished floors, especially if they are wearing footwear with smooth soles. It is also easy to trip over edge strips where there are changes in flooring materials. Unfortunately, single steps are often present at seating booths, seating areas, platforms, podiums, and stages. When someone stands up to leave a raised booth or raised seating area, a momentary lack of awareness and the tendency to look ahead rather than down at the floor can result in a fall.

Chapter 7

Stairways: Tumbling to the Bottom

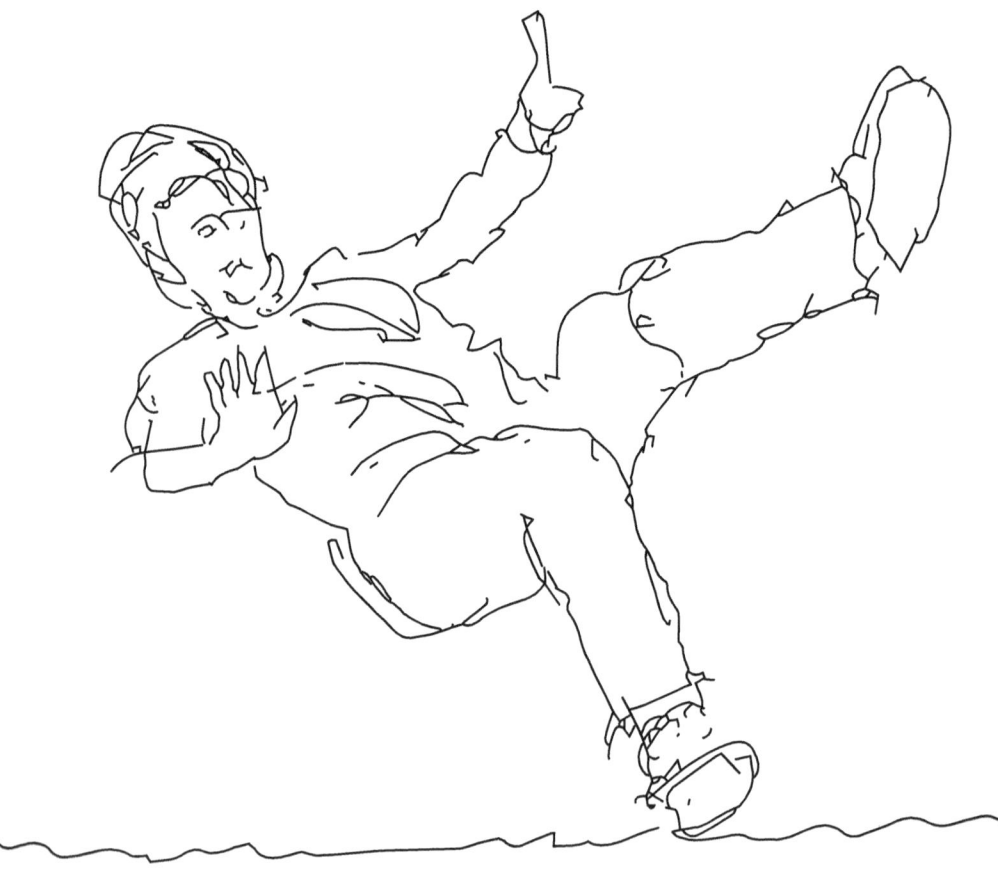

Stairway falls in public exterior and interior spaces are a major problem in our society, resulting in much unnecessary pain, suffering, and expense. Think about how people sometimes behave on stairs. Some people run up stairways taking two steps at a time and fly down them with great confidence. Teenagers and young adults do amazing acrobatics with skateboards as they jump onto handrails and sail to the bottom, sometimes wiping out, but seldom getting hurt, as they get back up and search out more challenging stairways. People are testing their limits all the time on stairs, and some people are used to flying around on stairways and feeling perfectly safe doing so.

However, when people have reduced vision, health problems, are carrying things, get distracted, or over-step their limits, they often get into trouble on stairs.

Too Many Stairway Falls

Hospital emergency room records throughout the country prove that falls on stairways are commonplace. In the United States more than 1 million people are injured, and more than 12,000 people die from stairway falls each year. Stairway injuries are the second leading cause of injury, behind motor vehicle injuries (National Safety Council, Injury Facts). John Templer, author of The Staircase, Studies of Hazards,

Falls, and Safer Design has referred to stairs as "the most dangerous consumer product in history" (Today Show Interview 10-3-96). CBS News reported that a child under the age of five falls down stairs, and is rushed to the hospital, every six minutes, on average.

You can hit your head and have a concussion, break bones, tear muscles or ligaments, hurt your back, or snap your neck from falling down a stairway. Poor design, poor construction and/or insufficient lighting can increase your chances of falling on stairs. Inattention, hurrying, tiredness, illness, dizziness, and the side effects of medications, drugs and alcohol can also contribute to your chances of falling and getting injured on stairs.

People expect stairways to be safe to use, and property owners have an obligation to inspect and maintain stairways, and to eliminate hazards that exist. But when someone falls down a stairway and files a lawsuit, the question is always "Who is negligent and to what extent?"

Most people do not fully understand the biomechanics of a fall on a stairway, or exactly what happens when a person unintentionally becomes airborne. Just as walking along a route is a flowing rhythmical movement, walking up or down a stairway is also rhythmical. But walking up and down stairways is more complicated than walking on a flat surface, and falls from stairs are often more serious because people typically fall greater distances.

Stair Components and Code Requirements

A stairway includes stairs, landings, and handrails. A landing is a flat level platform that is present at the top of stairs, at the bottom of stairs, and between flights of stairs. Flights of stairs are continuous stairs that are not interrupted by landings, so a stairway with one intermediate landing has two flights of stairs. The riser is the vertical part of a stair, and the tread is the horizontal part of a stair. Although unsafe situations are more prevalent in older, existing stairways, one should not assume that all new stairways are completely safe. Abnormalities at the top of stairways, abnormalities at the bottom of stairways, missing or loose handrails, handrails that are not continuous for the full length of the stairway, and handrails that do extend beyond the top and bottom of the stairway are all common problems, sometimes even on newer stairways.

Building codes, building code handbooks, industry standards, and research on stairway falls all give credence to the importance of having proper handrails on stairways. Handrails serve an important function by providing something for a person to hold onto and maintain balance while ascending and descending a stairway. They also provide something for people to grab onto when they misstep or start to fall, although there is precious little time to react once a person loses their balance. It is much safer to hold onto a handrail to prevent a fall in the first place, rather than trying to grab a handrail to stop the act of falling.

Both the International Building Code (IBC) and the ADA Standards require handrails to be continuous to the top and bottom of all stairways. Handrail extensions at the top of the stairs are required for safety because they allow people to secure their footing on the landings at the top of stairs before they step into the stairway. Handrails are required to have gripping profiles within specified parameters regarding dimensions and shapes, so that people can wrap their fingers around handrails to gain and maintain support. Without a proper gripping profile, it can be very difficult to obtain a secure hold of a handrail.

State-of-the-art building codes prohibit stair risers greater than seven inches high, and also require treads to be at least eleven inches long. This is to prevent stairways from being too steep, since steep stairways are known to be unsafe. Unfortunately, stairways in many older buildings were built with risers greater than seven inches and treads less than eleven inches, and basement stairways are often extremely steep.

Types of Stairway Falls

In Chapter Two I discussed the most common types of missteps that lead to falls that I have investigated during my career. A fall typically happens immediately after one of these types of events, when a person loses their balance. In addition to the most common types of missteps, stairway falls also include a 'heel-scuff', when the back of a person's shoe scuffs the riser of a stair (typically where there are short treads) and an 'under-step', when a person walking upstairs fails to get adequate footing on a stair tread. However, heel-scuffs and under-steps are not as common as other types of miss steps, and I have not investigated any falls when a heel-scuff or an under-step was determined to be the cause of a fall.

When I investigate a falling incident on a stairway, after someone missteps and falls, it is not always possible to determine with absolute certainty (unless there is clear video evidence of the falling event), which type of misstep occurred. However, if the person who fell was descending a steep stairway with short treads it is likely that an over-step occurred, and if the person fell while walking up a steep stairway it is likely that an under-step occurred. It is important to remember that using handrails for support makes falling on steep stairways less likely.

Abnormalities of Stairways

Stairway research at the National Bureau of Standards in the 1970s determined that seventy percent of stair accidents occur on the top three or bottom three stairs. Dimensional consistency of treads and risers within any flight of stairs is paramount for safety. Problems often exist at the top of stairs where the top riser is too high relative to the rest of the risers in the stairway. Although this can be the result of a lack of precision or proper detailing in the original construction, it often happens when hardwood flooring is added on to the floor at the top of a stairway. Whatever the cause, when the top riser in the stairway ends up being higher than the other risers in the stairway by more than 0.38in. (9.0mm), the stairway does not comply with the building code. Although 0.38in. (9.0mm) variation is the generally accepted tolerance, a variation of as little as 0.25in. (6.4mm) can initiate a trip or fall. Therefore, stairs should always be constructed with uniformly dimensioned treads and risers throughout.

Sometimes it is difficult to convince owners that an out of compliance stairway may be hazardous. One time I was completing a building assessment and was standing at the bottom of the stairway looking up at the top of the stairway while the building supervisor was standing next to me. I was having difficulty convincing him that the top riser was a safety hazard because it was higher than the other risers in the stairway. I recommended that he reconstruct the top of the stairway, and he said, "well, it has always been that way, and no one has ever fallen." Then, while we were standing there looking up the flight of stairs, a lady walking up the stairway in front of us caught the toe of her shoe on the edge of the top riser and fell forward onto the floor. Fortunately, she was not seriously injured, but she was shaken and bruised.

I thought that the chances of this happening while we were standing there were about the same as getting struck by lightning. But as I reflected on it later, I realized that the odds were not as great as I originally thought. It was predictable that people would catch the toes of their shoes on the top riser since it was more than one inch higher than the other risers in the stairway. In any case, after I had struggled to find the right words to convince the building supervisor, when he saw the woman trip and fall forward onto the floor, he became completely convinced that the top of the stairway was unsafe. Within a week he hired a carpenter to rebuild the top of the stairway and install new handrails with extensions.

Another stairway fall that I remember well occurred in a century-old building on the campus where I teach. The building was recently restored and rehabilitated, but for many years before the restoration it had an interior stairway with a short riser on the bottom stair. The basement of the building housed the university's photographic services department, which was a place that I visited on a regular basis. Every time I went down the stairway it bothered me that the bottom riser was noticeably shorter than the rest of the risers in the stairway, and I often stumbled over the last step onto the floor. One day I saw that a friend of mine who was an employee of photographic services had his arm in a cast. I asked, "What happened to you?" He said he was embarrassed to admit it, but he missed the bottom step and fell to the floor, breaking his arm in the process. He went on to say that he had walked down the stairway hundreds of times before without incident. When I told him that the bottom of the stairway was unsafe and did not comply with the current building code, he replied that it was his fault for not paying attention.

Falling Down Stairways

One evening after dark Zachery Jazzman was helping his daughter set up tables and decorations for her wedding reception in a meeting house in a small midwestern town. Zach had never been in the building before and was unfamiliar with the interior spaces, so when he needed to use the restroom, he walked towards a restroom sign that he saw mounted above an open doorway. The doorway was dark, so as he stepped into it, he felt around on the wall to find the light switch. As he did so he inadvertently stepped into an open stairway. There was no door or railing present at the top of the stairway and Zach tumbled all the way to the bottom, hitting his head and suffering a serious traumatic brain injury during his fall.

Zach's attorney asked me to inspect the location. I arrived at the building and took measurements, photos and light readings inside the doorway at the top of the open stairway. With the stairway light off, as it was when Zach fell, my light readings on the floor surface at the top of the stairs were all less than 0.1 foot-candle (1.09 lumens), or well below the minimum safe lighting level for a stairway.

Zach said in his deposition that he had no idea there was an open stairway inside the doorway, and that he thought he was entering the men's restroom. He also stated that it was very dark, and he couldn't see anything when he stepped inside the doorway. Zach's eyes would have gradually adjusted to a lower lighting level, but when he walked from the brightly lit space into the dark space, his eyes did not have enough time to adequately adjust to the lower lighting level. Zach essentially took an airstep into the open stairway as he tried to locate the light switch. The meeting hall was an old building that was constructed in the 1920s when there was no building code, so there were no building code violations that I could cite, even though the stairway would not have complied with the current building code. However, my research determined that the stairway did not comply with the state's Life Safety Code because of inadequate lighting.

The case went to trial and I testified that the location where Zach fell was unsafe and hazardous, that the lighting in the stairway did not comply with the state's Life Safety Code, and that the building owner was negligent for not providing a safe environment for the public. I also testified that the lighting on the floor at the top of the stairs where Zach fell was well below the minimum acceptable lighting level for safety and that the owner had a responsibility to keep the light on in the stairway at all times when the building is open, especially when passage down the stairway was the only way to get to the men's restroom.

Although I did not hear the defense's argument, they undoubtably claimed that Zach was negligent for walking into a dark unfamiliar area and not paying attention to his surroundings. They likely also argued that there were no code violations because it was a hundred-year-old building. Unfortunately for Zach, the jury ruled that he was more negligent than the building owner, and he received no financial compensation.

Zach's case would have been stronger if his attorney had been able to show actual building code violations which would have established "negligence per se," and that might have swayed the jury. I frankly don't understand why the jury ignored the Life Safety Code and was not more sympathetic to the inadequate lighting issue, but the meeting hall was in a small town in a rural Midwestern state where jurors often sympathize with small business owners and non-profit organizations rather than individuals who fall.

When I heard about the outcome of the trial I was surprised and disappointed because I had compassion for Zach who will have to live with the long-term impact of the traumatic brain injury he suffered during his fall. It is best not to assume that you will succeed in a lawsuit, even when there is some negligence on the part of the owner. I would like to go back to the building to see if they have made any safety and lighting improvements.

Doris Brown fell near the bottom of a concrete stairway in front of her church, landed on the sidewalk, and broke her wrist. When I met Doris' attorney at the church, I realized immediately that the stairway did not comply with building code because the handrails did not extend to, or beyond, the bottom of the stairway.

My inspection also revealed that the stair treads all had excessive slopes downward ranging between three and five percent, exceeding the maximum two percent slope allowed for drainage. An additional problem was that the stairs treads were shorter than the required eleven-inch minimum, making the stairway too steep. And finally, the bottom stair riser was shorter than the other stair risers.

The unsafe conditions made it very understandable why Doris fell while descending the stairway. The stairway was too step, the stair treads sloped forward, the bottom riser was hazardous, and the handrail did not extend to, or beyond, the bottom of the stairway. In my report I referenced my photos and measurements and the International Building Code (IBC) and ADA Standards. I also stated that it is common practice to paint the leading edges of the stair treads to make them more visible and increase safety, especially on the top and bottom of the stairs. The case was settled favorably for Doris before trial.

Mildred Miller was an active member in her church and was going downstairs to the fellowship hall when she fell to the bottom and broke her arm and shoulder. She hired an attorney who called me and explained the circumstances of her fall. After he described the stairway to me, I responded that the stairway likely had safety issues that contributed to her fall.

When Mildred's attorney and I met at the site, a church member met us to let us inside. He did not seem very happy to see us, and I sensed some hostility on his part. I carefully documented the location where Mildred fell. There were several unsafe conditions and building code violations, including an excessively steep stairway with short stair treads, a handrail on only one side of the stairs, the lack of an adequate gripping profile on the handrail, loose fitting carpeting on the stairs, and low lighting levels.

At trial I testified that Mildred likely over-stepped a stair tread on the steep stairway, and I elaborated about the handrail, loose carpeting, and low lighting. The defense argued that when the building was constructed, the church was exempt from being required to follow the building code. Mildred's attorney argued that there was no exemption for churches, and the building code did indeed apply. I then went on to describe the specific building code violations that were in effect when the church was constructed. The jury decided that Mildred was more negligent than the church was, and Mildred did not receive any financial compensation for her injuries.

The burden of proof is always on the plaintiff, and one could say that the defendant is presumed innocent until proven guilty. Even though the plaintiff identified unsafe conditions and actual building code violations, it was not enough to convince the jury that the church was more negligent than Mildred was. It should also be noted that, in this particular case, jurors were not sympathetic to one of the church members suing her own church.

Although Doris Brown also sued her own church, the plaintiff's attorney in that case was able to settle the dispute using the argument that there were three undisputed building code violations that constituted 'negligence per se'. The settlement may also have been made easier to achieve because the financial demand was lower and more reasonable.

In another case I was asked to investigate a fall down a stairway in a funeral home. William Harris was attending a wake service in a chapel addition to a historic house that had been a family-owned funeral business for many years. The fall occurred after William viewed the body of his friend and then turned to walk to the seating area in the back of the chapel. Unfortunately, he walked directly into an open stairway with no door or gate. William fell to the bottom of the stairway, hit his head, broke an arm, and dislocated his shoulder. In his deposition William said the lighting was very subdued in the chapel, and that he thought he was walking down an aisle and not a stairway. The stairway led to a room in the basement where caskets were on display for viewing and purchase.

William's attorney and I met at the funeral home where I took measurements, photos, and light intensity measurements with the lighting level set the same as when he fell. The lighting level at the top of the stairway was below 0.1 foot-candle (1.09 lumens), which was well below the minimum lighting level recommended by the lighting industry. There were no lights on in the stairway itself and dark carpeting on the floor continued down the stairway. In my report I described each unsafe condition including low walls along the sides of the top of the open stairway that made it look like an aisle rather than a stairway, no door or gate at the top of the stairway, handrails that did not extend to the top of the stairway, low lighting levels in the chapel, no lighting in the stairway itself, and the dark carpeting that continued down the stairway. I said that the stairway was easy to misread as an aisle due to a combination of these factors. I also explained that another factor may have been that William's eyes had not had time to fully adjust to the dark interior space when he fell.

At trial, the jury determined that the funeral home was more negligent than William was, and he was financially compensated for his injuries. The owners of the funeral home were upset with the jury's decision, but defendants are never pleased when a jury finds them to be responsible.

Denise Vaughn fell while walking up a stairway in a house that had a basement converted into a beauty salon. After visiting the salon, Denise walked up the stairs to leave. She was using the handrail, which was to her right, but the handrail was not continuous to the top of the stairs, so it was necessary for her to let go of it in order to reach ahead and grab a small handle that was mounted on the wood doorframe at the top of the stairs. As Denise attempted to reach for the handle, she lost her footing, fell backwards down the stairway, and suffered severe injuries.

Denise's attorney sent me photos, an explanation of the circumstances of her fall, measurements, and other pertinent information. I could see right away that it was clearly an unsafe stairway. In my report I identified five conditions in the stairway that were not in compliance with the building code and the ADA Standards: 1) there was a handrail on only one side of the stairway, 2) the handrail was not continuous to the top of the stairs, 3) the handrail did not have a proper profile for gripping, 4) the cabinet style handle that was mounted on the door frame at the top of the stairs was small, difficult to grab hold of, and was not a substitute for a proper handrail, and 5) the risers were greater than seven inches and the treads were less than ten inches, which made the stairway very steep.

Since the beauty salon business was in the basement of what had originally been a single-family residence, the existing stairway had been constructed under more lenient building code requirements. Older versions of building codes also allowed residential stairways to be steeper than stairways in public and commercial buildings, and only one handrail was required when the house was constructed. The defense could have argued that the older building code was the only code that applied. However, when the basement became a business that was open to the public, the owner had an obligation to upgrade the stairway to reasonable safety standards. The case settled before going to trial, and Denise received financial compensation for her medical expenses and injuries.

Handrails and Guardrails

Jill Farnham fell and broke her arm while walking down a stairway in her apartment building that had a loose handrail that pulled away from the wall while she was holding on to it.

I met Jill's attorney at the apartment building and observed that the anchoring supports for the handrails were lag bolts screwed into the stairway walls that had loosened over time and were no longer securely fastened. The loose handrail was essentially another hazard waiting for someone to find it. The handrail did not comply with the building code or the ADA Standards regarding handrail height, handrail extensions, and gripping profile. These additional unsafe conditions may have contributed to Jill's fall. My brief report and Jill's account of what happened was all that was needed for Jill's attorney to settle the case before trial.

Peter Larson was a blind man in his thirties who fell over a low railing into a stairwell in a century-old building. Peter was a short-term resident in the building that had been purchased by the state and converted into a facility to help rehabilitate people who were learning to cope with severe visual disabilities or blindness. The building had both overnight rooms and training rooms.

On the night he fell Peter had been drinking at a local bar. He returned to the building, went up to his room, got into his night clothes, and walked out of the room to go to the restroom. In order to get to the restroom Peter needed to walk past an open stairwell but when he did, he walked directly into a low railing and toppled over it. A sighted person would have seen the railing and turned left. Peter fell seventy feet and landed feet first on a terrazzo floor. He miraculously survived the fall but suffered severe fractures in both legs that required multiple surgeries and a long recovery. Amazingly, Peter was able to walk again, but with almost constant pain.

I was hired by the defense attorney for the state that owned the building, but I could not help but feel compassion for Peter and all his pain and suffering. When I arrived at the building, I measured the height of the guardrail as being just under 36in. (0.91m) high. The fact that the guardrail was 6.0in. (0.15m) lower than what current codes allowed, concerned me because, by today's standards, it was an unsafe condition.

During the next few days I researched building code requirements for guardrails. I confirmed that the current building code requires a minimum height of 42in. (1.1m). Another common problem is that older building codes required a minimum guardrail height of only 36in. (0.91m). Therefore, the guardrail in question would not comply with the current code, but since the building had been constructed in the early 1900s when there was no building code, there was no code violation.

For many years the minimum guardrail height was 36in. (0.91m), but people have gotten taller over the years, and building code authors have responded by raising the minimum guardrail height to 42in. (1.1m). Peter was 6ft. 4in. (1.93m) tall, which put him in the 97th percentile of height, so his center of gravity was above the top of the low guardrail that he fell over.

I called the state's attorney and reported that building codes are typically 'grandfathered'. In other words, the stricter requirements of the current building code are not retroactively applied to the older building. I said that I would be happy to testify at trial, but that if asked, I would be compelled to admit that by today's standards, the low guardrail is an unsafe condition. The day before I was to testify at trial, the state's attorney called me and told me that the case had been settled to both parties' satisfaction. I was surprised that the case resolved without a trial, but I suspect that Peter did not want to go to trial because he worried that because he had been drinking before he fell, the jury would be less sympathetic. It is also likely that Peter did not want to go through the stress and ordeal of a trial. During the phone call I strongly recommended that new guardrails be installed around the open stairwell, and eventually they were.

All building owners have an obligation to ensure that their buildings are safe for the public. Building code requirements are minimum requirements that often do not always reflect the state of the art, or best practice. Although building code authors knew that the 36in. (0.91m) guardrail height was too low, it took many years to get a consensus of voting members to upgrade the building code to require the 42in. (1.1m) minimum height.

Another common problem is that too many stairways have no handrails. Grand stairways and curved stairways with no handrails are often seen on television game shows, talk shows, and award ceremonies. One or two stairs without handrails are also typical at speaker's platforms and stages. While stairways without handrails are common and may or may not comply with the building code, they do not, in my opinion, represent good practice. Apparently actors, politicians, and set and theater designers think that having stairs is a sign of strength, and that handrails are a sign of weakness. Or maybe they think handrails distract from the elegance of the venues. However, while many people feel safe without handrails being present, others do not. Handrails do not need to be awkward looking or ugly. Instead, they can be beautifully designed elements that integrate seamlessly with stairway designs. Handrails should be thought of as essential for safety, and not as optional. Elegant and graceful solutions are needed, and handrails should be thought of as design opportunities rather than obnoxious after-thoughts.

Safe Use of Stairways

- Remember that you have a responsibility to arrive safely at the top or bottom of the stairway
- Stay aware and take care on every stair
- Be present at all times
- Always proceed with caution, and stay aware of your risk of falling
- Focus on walking safely up and down stairways
- Use extra caution and go slower when going down a stairway
- Be careful not to excessively over-step the edge of the stair when going down stairways
- Be careful not to catch the toe of your shoe on the edge of the stair when going up stairs
- Be aware of unsafe conditions on exterior stairs, including wet conditions, snow and ice covering, wet leaves or debris
- Consciously avoid distracting yourself or letting conversations distract you

- Tell yourself you don't need to save a few seconds by running, hurrying, or skipping stairs
- Make allowance for the side effects of medications
- Be extra careful if you have consumed alcoholic beverages
- Watch out for uneven steps, especially at the top and bottom of stairways
- Make it a habit to always use the handrail
- Keep one hand free to use the handrail when carrying items
- Be extra cautious when no handrails are present
- Do not block your vision of the stairs with items you are carrying
- Limit talking to others while using stairs
- Use your phone, tablet, or computer where it is safe to do so, but not while using stairs
- When distractions are unavoidable, minimize your risk by going slower and holding on to the handrail

Takeaways
There was no railing - but it contributed to my failing

A disproportionally high percentage of falls occur on stairways, and stairs can be killers, so people should not make falls more likely by behaving carelessly. Most stairway falls occur at the top or bottom of stairways, especially when the top or bottom riser is taller or shorter than the rest of the risers in the stairway. Older stairways in public buildings, and residential stairways, are often dangerously steep with short treads that are easy to over-step while descending. Stairways that do not have gripable handrails, or continuous handrails, and/or handrails on both sides are more dangerous. Refer to *Access for Everyone* for stairway illustrations, details, and recommendations.

Chapter 8
Moving Devices: Staying Alert

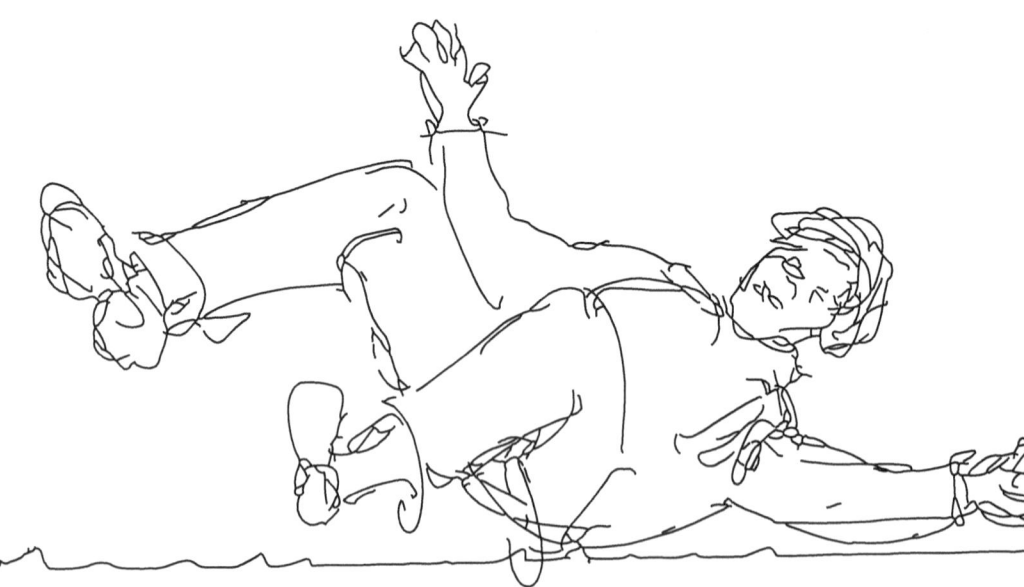

Falling on Moving Devices

Falls involving elevators, escalators, and moving walkways are not common, but they do happen. The Consumer Product Safety Commission reports that approximately 30 people die, and 17,000 people are seriously injured each year as a result of elevator and escalator incidents; so it is important not to let your guard down or assume that these devices are always completely safe. Equipment malfunction accounts for a small percentage of accidents, with careless behavior usually being the primary culprit, so people should always stay alert when using mechanical conveyances.

Elevators

Charlotte Brown fell while entering an elevator in a library. Charlotte was carrying several books in her arms as she stepped into the elevator. The door was in the open position, but she did not realize the elevator cab floor was a few inches lower than the floor level. When Charlotte stepped forward, she unknowingly took an airstep, fell forward, hit her head and suffered traumatic brain injury.

Her attorney sent me a surveillance video that showed the sequence of events that led up to and included Charlotte's fall. It showed two elevator repair men who were working on the elevator before she arrived, but they both walked away, presumably to get a tool or part. While they were away Charlotte did not know that the elevator was being serviced, although when she arrived at the elevator, the door was standing in the open position. The video showed her placing her foot forward into the elevator cab, taking an airstep, and falling forward as her body twisted. Her vision was partially blocked by the books she was carrying, and it was evident from her behavior that she was not aware of the fact that the floor level of the elevator cab was a few inches below the building floor level. In my report I articulated my analysis of Charlotte's fall and said that the elevator repair men were negligent for failing to either stay by the elevator and tell people it was not working or putting up yellow warning tape across the front of the open elevator cab before they walked away.

A settlement was reached, and Charlotte received financial compensation for her traumatic brain injury without having to go through a trial.

Moving Walkways
Most people walk at a pace of 2.5 mph (4.0 kmph) to 3.0 mph (4.8 kmph) and the average speed of a moving walkway is about the same speed. So when you walk on and off a moving walkway, you experience a sudden change, either doubling your speed or cutting it in half. Falls are more common when getting off moving walkways than when getting on them because people tend to pay careful attention when they get on, but once on the moving walkway they tend to relax and may forget how fast they are going.

I have investigated several falls where people fell off of the ends of moving walkways in an airport. In each case there was evidence that the user's behavior contributed significantly to the fall. One woman who fell was standing backwards and talking to someone, not realizing that she was at the end of the moving walkway. Even though she was holding on to the rubber side rail, she lost her footing and fell. Another woman was talking on a cell phone and not paying attention when she got to the end of the moving walkway, and a man fell off the end while running to catch a plane. Because he was running he was not prepared for the rapid deceleration that he experienced when he arrived at the end, and he stumbled and fell. Low lighting at the end of the moving walkways may have contributed to the falls, but inattention was the biggest factor. Each of the cases I investigated was settled before going to trial.

I was working for the defense in each of these cases and I was eventually able to make recommendations to the owner regarding improvements in lighting and other issues. I was pleased to see that my recommendations were followed and that moving walkways in several locations are now safer as a result.

Escalators

Most falls on escalators occur while getting on or off, and there is usually human error, inattention, or misjudgment involved. This is not to say that design errors, lighting, and equipment malfunctions are not possible; it is just that they are uncommon and unlikely. Individuals with balance or coordination issues are more likely to experience problems getting on and off escalators.

Using Caution on Moving Devices

- Stay alert and aware of your surroundings when you use an elevator, moving walkway, or escalator
- Look down before you step on and off elevators, escalators, and moving walkways
- If you are distracted, looking at your phone, are carrying items, and/or dragging suitcases, you are increasing your risk of falling on escalators and moving walkways
- If you are wearing a long skirt or coat, loose clothing or a scarf on an escalator, be especially careful (or use the elevator) since these items have been known to catch in the moving parts of escalators
- If you are hesitant to get on an escalator, take the elevator instead
- If you have dizziness or balance problems, use the elevator rather than the escalator

Takeaways
I shoulda paid attention - but now I am on my pension

Modern mechanical conveyance systems are, for the most part, safe and reliable, and equipment malfunctions are rare. However, to avoid falling, users should always be observant and exercise caution when getting in and out of elevators and on and off of escalators and moving walkways.

Chapter 9

Hazardous Homes: Where Most Falls Happen

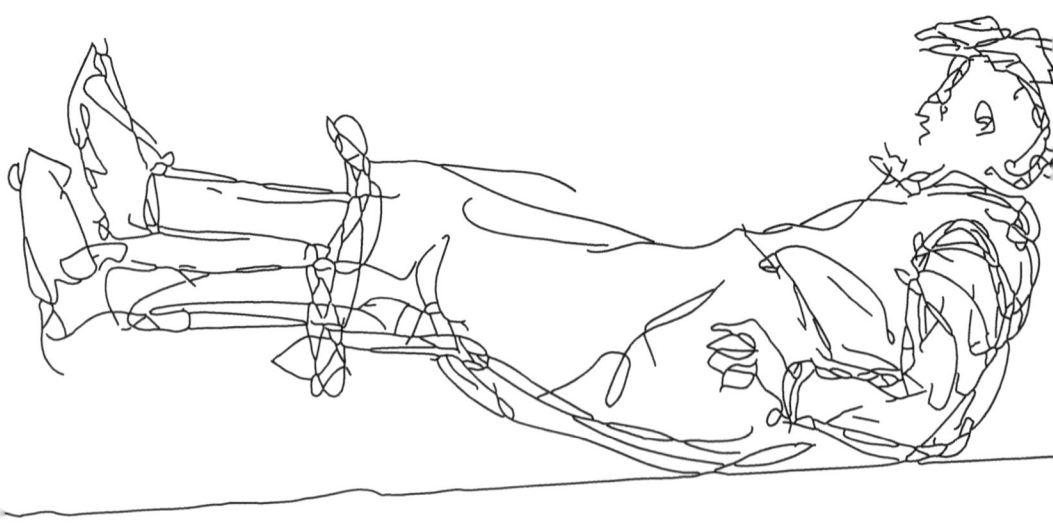

Too Many Falls at Home

The National Council on Aging estimates that more than three quarters of all falls in the United States take place either inside a home, or in close proximity to a home (NCOA website). Each year more than 900,000 children under the age of five are taken to emergency rooms for a stair related injury. This equates to once every six minutes, on average. Stairways are also the number one cause of injury for one-year-old children (The New York Times, 3/12/12). Older people are also more likely to fall down stairways in their own homes, resulting in too many unnecessary and avoidable injuries and death.

You are more likely to fall in your own home than in a public building or anywhere else, and yet I have had few cases involving falls in private residences. I suppose this is because homeowners don't have a way to sue themselves for being negligent, and if they did, they would have to pay for both lawyers' fees! I have had a few cases where guests in private residences fell and sued the homeowners. However, it is difficult to convince a jury that the homeowner is negligent, and it certainly does not foster a warm friendship between owner and guest.

There are many reasons why our homes present the biggest fall hazards. First of all, most of us spend most of our time at home. Secondly, we tend to accept having obstacles on the floor, poor lighting, throw rugs, and other hazards.

Housing Sites and Driveways

When it comes to fall safety for single family homes, common sense seems to have been thrown out the window. Far too many houses are constructed with excessively steep and hazardous driveways. For people making deliveries and for friends and family who come to visit, parking in the street in front of the house and walking up those driveways is often the only option to get to the front door. Sometimes there are walks and stairs leading up to the houses, but they are usually too steep and/or have no handrails.

Postal delivery people often have to travel up and down steep driveways, hazardous walks, stairs without handrails, and then step onto porches or landings to get to home owner's mailboxes five days a week. Now that we have UPS, FedEx, Amazon, pizza delivery, meals on wheels, etc., the problem has been multiplied.

Prudent planning and design strategies are needed. Developers and home builders should site houses and grade around them appropriately to avoid having dangerously steep routes and driveways. Home buyers would be wise to think about these issues when selecting and buying their houses.

Visitability

For people who have trouble using stairs and those who cannot negotiate stairs at all, the vast majority of single family homes are full of unnecessary obstacles. 'Visitability' is a concept that is being promoted for the design of single family homes that is much needed but unfortunately is very atypical. Visitability features include:
- at least one no step entrance,
- wider doors and hallways,
- a bathroom on the first floor (preferably an accessible bathroom with an accessible shower),
- bathroom walls that are reinforced for the installation of grab bars,
- light switches and electrical outlets that are mounted at the appropriate reachable heights, and preferably a bedroom (or other room that can be converted to a bedroom) on the first floor.

These features facilitate aging in place while increasing safety, and yet few houses are constructed with them.

A few communities around the country have mandated that a small percentage of single family houses be designed and constructed with at least some visitability features. However, if you try to find a house in your community that has grade level access and a no-step entrance, you will likely be very disappointed. You can help promote visitability by advocating for it with your civic leaders and city council.

Slipping Hazards

Slipping on a kitchen floor is easy to do. You might ignore the liquid spills or splatters on the floor and wait for them to dry up. Why do you accept this in your own home when you expect the staff in the grocery store to clean up their spills right away? Since most falls happen in the home, it is a good idea to replace smooth, slippery, and worn out floor materials with new slip-resistant materials and, to further reduce your chances of slipping and falling in the kitchen, do not use cleaning and waxing products that make floors slippery.

The bathroom is probably the most hazardous room in your house, but it doesn't need to be. Start by examining your bathrooms to identify any potential slipping hazards such as smooth floors and tub bottoms. When your floors get wet do they also get slippery? Some bathroom flooring materials are much more prone to becoming slipping hazards than others. Analyze your tub and shower floor surfaces because you may find that it would be a good time to upgrade them. It may also be a good time to install grab bars on walls next to toilets and in tubs and showers. When we remodeled two bathrooms in our house recently, we lined all the walls with thick plywood before installing drywall and tile so we would have solid blocking to securely mount grab bars wherever we needed them. Then we installed two grab bars in each shower, a horizontal grab bar on the wall, and a vertical grab bar near the head of the shower for getting in and out. We also added grab bars next to the toilets where towel bars are often placed so that we have something solid to hold and push up on, should we or any of our guests ever need them. Towel bars are not reliable or secure enough to support your weight, and they are no substitute for properly anchored grab bars that are designed to support at least 250 lbs (1112 N) of force. A towel bar is designed to support a couple of towels so don't install a towel bar where you should install a grab bar. I purchased high quality grab bars that fully meet safety standards but do not have an institutional appearance, so they do not negatively impact the aesthetics of bathrooms.

Stairways

For years I have enjoyed looking at publications featuring great housing. They often include fabulous photos of beautifully designed stairways, but it continually amazes me how many stairways that are featured do not have handrails. Often these sweeping stairways are curved with open risers that seem to magically float in space. Otherwise mediocre interior spaces are brought to life with these masterpieces of design, engineering, and construction. They look incredible and many users obviously go up and down them without falling, or fear of falling. However, I wonder what happens when parents and grandparents come to visit and the guest rooms are located on the second floor, and what happens when the home owners get older and are not as steady on their feet as they used to be.

Probably the biggest reason people fall down their own stairways is because they let their guard down in their own familiar surroundings. Complacency kicks in and common sense rules don't seem to apply. Familiarity becomes your enemy when you lose your ability to discern danger.

When we visit other people's homes it is easy for us to see safety hazards, but when we walk through our own homes, it is easy for us to ignore them. In your own home, you tend to overlook unsafe conditions that are right in front of your eyes. You might see them, but you do not recognize them as hazards, or you rationalize that it is not that bad, or that it is too difficult to correct. You might say to yourself: "I know that step is too high, but I can adjust to it," and most of the time you do, but there is that one time when you do not. I know that light bulb at the top of the stairs is too small, but it has always been that way. I know I should install another handrail, but it is too difficult and expensive.

We are all susceptible to developing bad stairway habits. In our house I have set things on the bottom stair with the good intention of taking them upstairs later, but then I got lazy and walked around them rather than taking them to their intended destination. I have walked up and down a steep stairway without using the handrail, I have worn slippery socks and worn out footwear, and I have carried too much instead of taking several trips. I have neglected to turn the lights on before walking down dark basement stairs. Even though I know better, I admit that I have done all of these things in the past. I have known for years that these behaviors are risky, but I have rationalized that I was not at risk of falling because that happens to the 'other guy'. The reality is that sometimes I have ended up being that other guy. It may be easier not to change bad habits than it is to change them, but we could all end up as part of a statistic if we are not careful enough using stairs in our own homes.

A common hazard is a steep basement stairway that does not have adequate handrails, which is especially unsafe for people who go too fast and older people. After walking up and down the basement stairs with no handrails in our house for several years, I finally decided to install a good sturdy handrail. Since the stairway has an unusual configuration and a ninety degree turn, I could not use a standard handrail because it would require both turns and a vertical section of handrail. After thinking about it for a while I decided to configure a handrail with 1.5in. (38.1mm) inch diameter plastic PVC pipe and pipe connectors. Before long I assembled a custom handrail with a good gripping surface that was securely anchored to the walls. The new handrail is continuous and has two turns and a short vertical section that make it easy to grab, no matter where I am on the stairway. Now that I have the handrail in place I find that I use it all the time, even though I was once convinced that I did not really need it. Does this make my storage of items on one side of the basement stairs more acceptable? No, it does not; so I am working to change that bad habit as well.

Gabriel Cooper fell down a basement stairway at his friend's house. He was an overnight guest in the ranch style house and his bedroom was at the end of the hall. During the night he woke up and went into the kitchen to get a glass of water. When Gabe walked back towards the bedroom it was dark and he got turned around. He opened a door to the basement, thinking it was the door to his bedroom. He stepped into space, tumbled to the bottom of the stairs, breaking his arm and suffered a concussion and traumatic brain injury in the process. Gabe obtained the services of an attorney and filed a lawsuit against the homeowner, knowing full well that his friend had homeowner's insurance.

When I inspected the location there was no landing at the top of the stairs, just a door that swung into the top of the stairway. The house was built in a rural area outside of a small town where there was no building code enforcement. When the house was constructed, laws in the state did not require rural areas to comply with the building code, so even though there were several violations to the code, I could not cite them as code violations. Instead I described the unsafe conditions and explained why the stairway would not comply with the current code. The unsafe conditions included: no landing at the top of the stairway, no light at the top of the stairway, short stair treads and high stair risers that made the stairway steep, and only one handrail that did not extend to the top of the stairway.

The case went to trial and the defense argued that there were no building violations and that Gabe should have been aware of his surroundings and should have watched where he was going. In my testimony for the plaintiff I described the conditions in the stairway and explained why the stairway was unsafe. The jury found for the defense, and Gabe received no financial compensation for his medical expenses, lost wages, or pain and suffering. If the plaintiff had been able to pin down actual building code violations, the case might have settled before trial.

I don't know what went through the minds of the jurors, but I suspect they were not sympathetic to Gabe suing his friend. Additionally, jurors probably realized that his friend had homeowner's insurance, even though by law that cannot be disclosed during a trial. Jurors may have thought that Gabe was trying to exploit the deep pocket of the insurance company and did not want to set a precedent that could lead to higher insurance rates for all homeowners. Maybe Gabe and his attorney made a large financial demand that was seen as padded, or beyond what was reasonable. Sometimes jurors have great empathy for a person's injuries, pain, and suffering caused by a fall, but it may not be enough to convince them that the defendant was more negligent than the plaintiff.

Reduce Falls at Home
Assess and analyze your home
- Analyze the driveway and walks leading up to your house, and identify steep slopes and tripping hazards
- Measure the height from walks to front stoops and porches
- Learn how to recognize and correct falling hazards outside and inside
- Conduct a home safety assessment, or get professional help to do it
- Analyze all floor and stair surfaces to ensure they are firm, stable, and slip resistant
- Inspect transitions between flooring materials to ensure that there are no tripping hazards

Develop good habits
- Remember that you are most likely to fall in your own home or apartment, even though you are familiar with it
- Analyze the daily routines and habits that may be increasing your risk of falling
- Remember to stay alert and observant in your own familiar home environment

Improve driveways, walks, and exterior stairs
- Where appropriate, reroute and/or reconstruct driveways to achieve safe slopes

- If the height from the walk to the front stoop or porch exceeds 8.0in. (0.20m), reconstruct sections of the walk to reduce the height to 7.0in. (0.18m) maximum
- Eliminate tripping hazards in driveways and walks
- Fill hazardous gaps and cracks in driveways and walks
- Reconstruct hazardous exterior stairways
- Install handrails, with easy-to-grip profiles, on exterior stairs

Maintain areas outside
- Keep your entry, deck, stairs, and sidewalk clear of snow, ice, leaves, twigs, and debris
- Inspect your walks periodically and eliminate trippers, unsafe edges, and severe slopes
- Install low voltage lights that automatically turn on at dusk alongside the walk leading to your front door
- Ensure downspouts are placed so that water does not drain onto walking surfaces and freeze
- Seal cracks between sections of concrete walks and stoops or stairs where water can seep into cracks and cause settling or frost heave
- Repair or replace uneven pavement on sidewalks and driveways

Maintain the inside
- Choose sturdy furniture that has firm support and sturdy armrests that are safe to use
- Ensure that all existing furniture is structurally sound
- Rearrange furniture to ensure safe routes to, and around, furniture groupings
- Move coffee tables and other objects out of pathways
- Keep cabinet doors and drawers closed when not in use
- Keep hazardous dishwasher doors closed except when loading or unloading dishwashers

Eliminate tripping hazards
- Ensure that all transitions between floor materials are not tripping hazards

- Keep paths clear of obstacles such as shoes, purses, books, magazines, toys, and backpacks
- Keep the route from your bed to your bathroom clear of obstacles to ensure a safe trip to the bathroom in the middle of the night
- Move electrical cords and extension cords out of walking paths
- Install outlets where needed to avoid using extension cords
- Eliminate loose rugs and throw rugs
- Replace worn carpeting with dense, short pile carpeting
- Replace high thresholds at doors with low profile thresholds

Eliminate slipping hazards

- Reduce your chances of slipping in your kitchen and bathroom by cleaning up spills immediately
- Ensure you have adequate slip resistance on flooring and in tubs and showers
- Watch out for surfaces that become slippery when snow is tracked in and melts
- Replace slippery floor coverings with slip resistant no-wax materials
- Allow freshly mopped floors to dry before walking on them
- Be extra careful when using shampoos that make tub and shower floor surfaces slippery

Improve lighting and visibility

- Keep your entryways well lit
- Increase overall lighting for greater visibility
- Install additional lighting fixtures and lamps, and replace bulbs with brighter bulbs where appropriate
- Ensure that lighting is evenly distributed
- Install nightlights in bathrooms, bedrooms, and hallways where appropriate
- Install lighted switches in locations throughout your house where appropriate
- Keep flashlights in strategic places, such as nightstands, or use your cellphone's built-in light when needed

- Ensure that all stair edges are easy to see and well lit
- Eliminate or control glare by installing easy to operate window control devices and eliminating highly reflective surface materials
- Replace confusing patterned carpeting with low pile, solid colored carpeting

Install grab bars
- Install vertical and/or horizontal grab bars in appropriate locations in bathrooms, tub enclosures, shower stalls, and next to toilets, next to doorways, and in other locations in your home where needed
- Do not install towel bars where grab bars are needed, install grab bars instead
- Replace towel bars with grab bars where appropriate
- Ensure that all grab bars will support at least 250 lbs (1112 N) of force and are securely anchored

Behave cautiously on all stairways
- Always take care on every stair
- Stay alert when using stairs, and don't become complacent in your own familiar home
- In older homes, go slow, be careful, and always use the handrail, especially when using steep stairways and basement stairs
- Make a conscious effort to get solid footing on short stair treads and make sure that most of your foot lands squarely on each stair tread
- Rather than carrying heavy or large items, transfer items to smaller containers and take more trips with smaller loads
- Educate your children and grandchildren about the dangers of stairs, and instruct them on proper stair usage and the importance of using handrails
- Do not allow children to play on stairs or play with toys on stairs
- Avoid carrying children up and down stairs, but if you must, use the handrail and do not carry other items at the same time
- Keep stairs clean and clutter free

- Don't store items on the stairs
- Place items you intend to go up or down stairs in a basket with a handle and place the basket where it won't be an obstacle
- Turn on the lights when going up or down stairs when it is dark and when lighting is inadequate

Minimize stairway distractions
- Eliminate or remove distractions such as photos and paintings from stairway walls and at the top and bottom of stairways
- Remove mirrors from walls at the top and bottom of stairways, as people tend to look at their own reflections rather than concentrate on navigating the stairway

Inspect your stairways
- Check stairs for dimensional consistency, especially at the top and bottom of the stairway
- Inspect wood exterior stairs for structural integrity and excessive wear
- Inspect all exterior stairs for slippery surfaces
- Inspect handrails to ensure they are securely fastened, can support your entire body weight, and have proper gripping
- Inspect handrails to determine if they extend at least to the top and bottom of stairs
- Inspect stair coverings to ensure that they are tight and securely fastened
- Assess stairway lighting and switch locations to make sure they are adequate

Improve stair and deck safety outside
- Repair or replace stairs that do not have dimensional consistency
- Repair or replace excessively worn stairs
- Keep exterior stairs clear of snow, ice, leaves and debris
- Install low voltage lighting and timers to illuminate exterior stairs
- Remove slippery algae and lichens from wood stair treads, railings, and decks

Improve stair safety inside
- Ensure that you have easy-to-grip and secure handrails that extend at least the full length of the stairway
- To increase your safety, extend handrails beyond the top and bottom of stairs where appropriate
- Install sturdy safety railings at both the top and bottom of stairways
- Stain or paint handrails so that they have good contrast with the walls they are mounted on
- Use solid colors and avoid confusing patterns on stairs
- Make stair coverings a different color than floor coverings at the top and bottom of the stairways to make stairways more visible
- Install contrasting color strips along the leading edges of stairs where appropriate
- Ensure that all stair coverings are tightly fastened and hire a professional to replace or re-stretch loose carpeting on stairs
- If you install new carpeting on stairs, ensure that it is low pile, tight weave carpeting
- Remove loose mats or rugs at the top and bottom of stairs
- Ensure that all interior stairs have good lighting
- Maintain adequate lighting to make the leading edges of all stair treads visually legible
- Use matt finishes to avoid glare on stairs
- Install three-way light switches at the bottom and top of stairways
- Ensure that all stair treads have good slip resistance

When designing and constructing new stairways or rebuilding old stairways
- Design and construct stairways with young children and older people in mind
- Install sturdy handrails that have a gripping profile and proper extensions at the top and bottom of new stairways
- Construct intermediate landings when stairways have more than twelve risers

- Install sturdy gates that can safely swing open at the top and bottom of stairways
- Ensure that all treads and risers within the stairway have no more than 0.38in. (9.0mm) variation, and reconstruct stairs to make treads and risers dimensionally consistent where necessary
- When handrails are not present on both sides of stairways, install additional handrails
- If existing handrails are not easy to grip, replace them with easy-to-grip handrails
- Construct new stairs with risers no higher than 7.0in. (0.18m) and treads that are at least 11.0in. (0.28m) long
- Use non-glare stair treads and avoid using highly polished materials in stairways
- Use solid colored, uniformly textured, slip-resistant stair coverings
- Ensure that the color of handrails contrasts with the walls they are attached to
- Continue handrails around all intermediate stairway landings

Takeaways

What was I thinking - I should not have been drinking

People have the greatest risk of falling in their own home or apartment. Stairways, bathrooms, and kitchens are typically where most falls occur, but a fall can occur in any room or space. Just because you are familiar with your own living environment does not mean it is safe. It may be best to have an objective outsider with fresh eyes conduct a fall safety assessment, because you may not recognize many of the hazards that exist.

Chapter 10

After You Fall: What's Next?

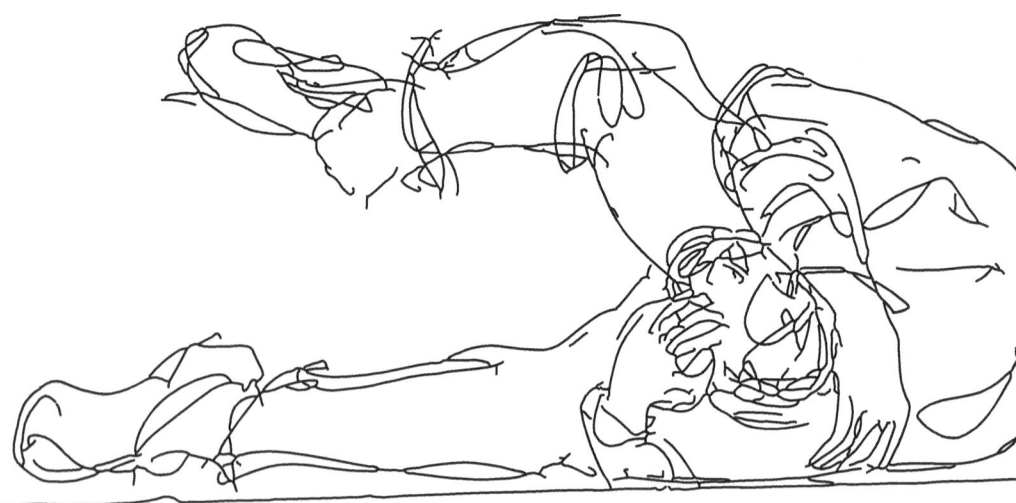

After You Fall

The first thing to do when you fall is to try and remain calm. There is no point in straining yourself or making heroic efforts to get up right away unless, of course, you are in harm's way. If you are badly injured call for help. If you determine it is safe to get up, do so with care. If you hit your head or suspect that you have any injuries at all, get medical attention as soon as possible. If you are taking blood thinners when you hit your head you could get dangerous bleeding, so see your doctor right away.

If you think you may have encountered a falling hazard and are considering consulting with an attorney, take photos, or have a friend or family member take photos of the location as soon as possible. Get close up photos of the exact location of your fall, but also get photos from farther back to show the context and the surroundings from different viewpoints. If you tripped on a hazard, photograph the vertical height of the tripping hazard while laying something flat like a book over the crack and holding a tape measure or ruler against the vertical edge to document the height from the lower surface to the upper surface. If you don't have a tape measure with you, use something to show scale, like a quarter or dollar bill, or a credit card.

If there were any witnesses, get their names, addresses, email addresses, and phones numbers, and if an accident report was made, ask for a copy. Keep in mind that medical records are important evidence that will help if you decide to seek compensation for your injuries. While it is fresh in your mind, write down and date your recollections of exactly what happened before, during, and after your fall. Note what you were carrying, what you were wearing, what kind of footwear you were using, where you were looking, what the weather was like, and other details to the best of your memory.

If an owner or manager speaks to you, be careful what you say and avoid admitting blame or negligence on your part if you are thinking of calling an attorney.

Living and Reliving Your Fall

It is exasperating when you fall and suffer injuries. If you are fortunate you may experience a full recovery, although that is often not the case. But regardless of your degree of recovery, you might find yourself reliving the fall in your mind and the "what ifs" over and over again. What if I had not been looking at my phone? What if I had not been wearing flip-flops? What if I had not been in a hurry? And if you blame others whom you think were negligent for leaving a spill on the floor or not fixing a crack in the sidewalk, you keep thinking about that as well. There is also the pain that comes back again when the weather changes or when you overexert yourself too much, and there is the unfortunate fact that once you fall, you may be more likely to fall again. This is especially true for people of advanced age and people with certain diseases or medical conditions.

However, if you take a case to trial you will likely relive the fall in excruciating detail, sometimes over and over again, in the form of phone calls and meetings with your attorney, talking to experts, giving testimony at a deposition, and at trial.

Should You File a Lawsuit?

If you fall where a hazardous condition existed, you have a right to sue the property owners because they have an obligation to identify hazards, to warn visitors of those hazards, and to correct them. So, naturally you may ask yourself, are others responsible or negligent, and do you have the right to be financially compensated for your injuries, medical expenses, pain and suffering, and lost wages? It is tempting to think that you are entitled to a huge financial reward. I read about a case in New York State where someone tripped and fell on an uneven sidewalk, suffered severe knee injuries, and received compensation worth over $2 million dollars. Although large amounts are possible, and do happen sometimes, my experiences usually tell a different story.

I have been a university professor in an architecture department for the past 40+ years and have been fortunate to be called on as an expert to investigate falls more than 350 times. I have completed investigations that have included research, analysis, and reports for both plaintiff and defense attorneys. Working for both the plaintiff and defense on different cases has helped me stay objective and fair minded. I have averaged about seven or eight investigations per year and the experiences and lessons learned have added up over time.

My investigations have increased my understanding of the roles that planning, design, construction methods, supervision during construction, management, and maintenance all have in making the built environment safe and free of hazards. Over the years I have been fortunate to engage in consulting activities, typically on weekends, breaks, and summers, without interfering with my teaching schedule or other responsibilities as a professor. The experiences have greatly enhanced my teaching in the form of case studies and specific examples that I have shared with students in the classroom.

I have also had more than 200 additional inquiries from attorneys about matters involving falls that were either dropped or not pursued after we discussed the merits of their potential cases. That represents a fairly high percentage of inquires that don't lead to compensation for people who fall. People who fall often find it difficult to find an attorney who will agree to represent them, and in many situations attorneys cannot find an expert who can make a credible argument to establish the defendant's negligence. A plaintiff's attorney needs to be convinced that there is negligence on the part of the owner or manager, and also needs to be able to line up the appropriate expert(s) to investigate and support that position.

Of the 350+ investigations that I have worked on, approximately 10% have ended up in the hands of a jury. In other words, 90% of the cases were either dropped or settled, with the vast majority being settled. Some, but not many, were resolved through mediation, a process that sometimes works in an effort to avoid a costly trial. Settlements were almost always compromises where neither side obtained what they started out wanting or ended up with what they thought they deserved. The plaintiff and the plaintiff's attorney start off trying to get full compensation for their demand, but unless both sides reach an agreement on a dollar amount, the case is probably headed for trial. Frequently the defense is not willing to offer financial compensation to settle the claim or offers a very low token amount. Then the plaintiff is left with the option of either dropping the matter or taking it to trial.

Suppose that the defense does not offer to settle, and you decide to take the matter to trial. When you fall and get hurt, you have the right to sue and you have a right to your day in court, but trials can be, and usually are, very stressful for the plaintiffs and their families. The defense knows this and is counting on it. I have seen several cases dropped or settled right before trial because the plaintiff got cold feet and did not want to appear at trial. In those cases, the plaintiff either got nothing or settled at the last minute for a token amount.

When you take your case to trial you also risk not getting any financial compensation at all. Juries are asked to determine if there was any negligence on the part of the plaintiff and the defense, and then they are charged with determining the percentage of fault of both sides. This is what is known as comparative fault. The comparative fault system is used in personal injury cases, including slip and fall cases, to award liability and damages based on the percentage of negligence of each party involved. There are negligence laws in all 50 states, but the laws vary from state to state. There are three types of systems;

comparative negligence, pure comparative negligence and modified comparative negligence.

Twelve states (Alaska, Arizona, California, Florida, Kentucky, Louisiana, Mississippi, Missouri, New Mexico, New York, Rhode Island, and Washington) use what is known as a pure comparative negligence system. In those states the court awards damages based on the percentage of fault of each party. If, for example, the plaintiff is found to be 80% negligent and the defense is found to be 20% negligent, the plaintiff can receive 20% of the amount determined by the court to be fair compensation. The pure comparative negligence system has been criticized because it allows a plaintiff who is primarily at fault to recover something from a defendant who is not primarily at fault. South Dakota has its own 'slight-gross' negligence system that is considered to be a modified pure comparative negligence system.

Five states (Alabama, Maryland, North Carolina, Virginia, and Washington, D.C.) have what is known as pure contributory negligence laws where the plaintiff cannot be awarded any financial damages if it is determined that the plaintiff has any degree of fault, even when it is as low as 1%. If, for example, the plaintiff is found to be 10% negligent and the defense is found to be 90% negligent, the plaintiff will not receive any compensation. Plaintiffs typically have a difficult time getting financial compensation for falls in those states.

The remainder of the states (the majority of states) have modified comparative negligence laws where each side (the plaintiff and the defense) is responsible for damages in proportions to their own percentage of fault, but only if the plaintiff's negligence is determined by the court to be less than either 50% or 49% (some states use the former, and the others use the latter, percentage). For example, if the plaintiff in any of these states is found to be 60% negligent, the plaintiff is not awarded any compensation. On the other hand if the defense is found to be 60% negligent, then the plaintiff will be awarded 60% of the amount determined by the court to be fair compensation. Check with your attorney to determine which type of negligence system is currently in place in your state.

Let us review a scenario of what could happen if you settle your case before going to trial in one of the states that has a modified comparative negligence law. After months of pleadings, interrogatories, and depositions, let's assume the defense is willing to settle an initial claim of $100,000 for $55,000 for compensation for medical care, recovering lost wages, and payouts for emotional distress. Let's assume that both sides agree to the figure based on the evidence, facts, and the concept of comparative fault. Then the attorney's fees are subtracted (typically based on a percentage of the settlement amount ranging from 30-40%). In our example, let us say the attorney's fee is 35%. That brings the amount down to sixty-five percent of $55,000, or $35,750. But the attorney will typically deduct the expenses paid for expert witness fees, filing fees, deposition fees, transcripts, trial exhibits, postage, etc. from that amount. Let's assume that those fees total $15,000. That brings the plaintiff's actual compensation amount down to $20,750. That may not sound like much money for all the months of pain, suffering, and anxiety. Sometimes the settlements are larger, but unfortunately settlement amounts are frequently small.

Taking your case to trial can be a risky proposition. Obviously the experience, skill level, and demeanor of your attorney make a big difference, but there are many other variables in a trial that affect the outcome. These include the strength of the evidence, the believability of the experts, the past experiences and attitudes of the jurors, and the judge's rulings. Consider these questions: do you have a credible expert that can articulate an unsafe condition in straightforward language that a jury will understand and relate to? Are there code violations? Does the location where you fell conform to industry standards? Was the owner negligent for not providing warning and/or not maintaining or repairing the unsafe condition? Will jurors sympathize with you, the property owner, or both? Will jurors like or dislike you, the way you look, the way you speak, and/or the way you dress? Will jurors be empathetic with your pain and suffering?

Juries often do not sympathize much with people who "do not watch where they are going." Some jurors might be thinking that they have all stumbled themselves and they didn't sue the property owners, so why should you get a windfall when they did not? After many years of experience as an expert witness, I am convinced of one thing: juries are unpredictable. I have seen strong cases for the plaintiff result in decisions for the plaintiff and strong cases for the defense result in decisions for the defense, but I have also worked on cases for the plaintiff when there was overwhelming evidence of code violations and unsafe conditions, but the jury decided for the defense and the plaintiffs received no financial compensation whatsoever. I have also seen decisions where the plaintiff's case had little or no merit, and yet the plaintiffs were awarded damages. However, in my experience this is rare. I am not advising not to take your case to trial, but if you do decide to proceed, you should do so with a full understanding of the risks and have a realistic expectation of what outcomes are possible.

There is a lot that goes on behind the scenes, and as an expert I never really get the full picture of the entirety of the case or what takes place in the courtroom or the jury room. Having served on a jury myself, I have a great respect for the jury process, and overall, I think it works pretty well. It is not a perfect system and it would benefit from some fine-tuning, but it appears to be as good or better as any other system that has been tried throughout history.

Positive change often occurs following judgments for the plaintiff when falling hazards are recognized and eliminated by property owners, and when staff are trained to maintain safe conditions at buildings and sites. Businesses have changed their policies, procedures, and training protocols following lawsuits, and codes and standards have been updated in important ways that make the built environment safer. New legal precedents have also resulted, following lawsuits involving falls.

One of the most satisfying elements of my work as an expert witness has been seeing the improvements that were made as a result of plaintiff's lawsuits. Many owners and managers have responded by making positive improvements to locations to eliminate falling hazards. Warnings have been added, tripping hazards have been corrected, guardrails have been installed, single steps have been eliminated, sidewalks with excessive cross-slopes have been replaced, handrails have been added, and grab bars have been installed. Whenever I have been able to, I have followed up with attorneys or revisited locations to determine if improvements were made.

Most of the time, owners and managers have acted on their own to eliminate falling hazards after going through settlement negotiations or trials, but it would be best if plaintiff's attorneys would insist on improvements as part of their demands and as part of settlement negotiations.

When I started my work as an expert witness, I made the commitment to myself to always be as objective as possible and not take sides with either the plaintiff or the defense. After all, it is up to the jury to hear both sides of the story, to listen to all the evidence, and to make the correct judgement. My job as expert is to conduct a thorough site inspection, to review and analyze the evidence, and state my informed opinion concerning the applicability of building codes, industry standards, and whether the location of the fall was safe or unsafe. I always find myself empathetic to anyone who falls and suffers injuries, but I do not let my empathy influence my opinion regarding safety issues or code compliance.

The Battle of the Experts

During the course of my career I have worked for attorneys on both sides, the plaintiff and the defense. This has helped me understand both points of view in each matter I research. The vast majority of my investigations started with a referral from another attorney, and several times an opposing attorney hired me later to work on another case. I always consider this to be a great compliment.

Sometimes I experience what is known as the battle of the experts, which happens when both sides hire experts. Since the burden of proof is on the side of the plaintiff, their expert produces the first report. Then the defense expert responds, often with a contradictory opinion. It has occurred to me that this is hypocritical because a hazard is a hazard and a code violation is a code violation. They should be indisputable, so why don't experts agree with each other? Is it right for experts to slant their opinions to help the side they are working for?

Sometimes this can be a moral dilemma for those of us who work on both sides of the fence. My approach has always been to be honest, no matter which side I represented. However, as I have learned to stay within the range of my own moral compass, I have also come to recognize that many situations are complex. To explain further the battle of the experts, I need to provide a bit more background regarding my research methodology.

By the time I have agreed to work for an attorney on a case, I have already expressed a preliminary opinion based on my review of photos and other information. I call the attorney and share my preliminary opinion before agreeing to accept payment to work on the matter. Many inquires I receive do not get pursued because my preliminary opinion does not adequately support the case.

Whether I am working for the plaintiff or the defense, I typically go through many of the same steps in my investigation. Let's review an example where I am asked by the defense to review an expert's report for the plaintiff. The report cites specific code violations, so I research them. If I agree that there are indeed code violations, I call the defense attorney and discuss the particulars. At that point the attorney may say, "I think we will try to settle this one without calling you as an expert, thanks for your preliminary analysis." Or, more commonly, the defense attorney will hire me and ask me to thoroughly review and analyze the report and other documents, point by point. If I find that the report includes vague generalities or unsupported statements, I will discuss that with the attorney who typically asks me to write a report with my findings. I typically state that my opinion is preliminary and subject to change if additional relevant information comes forward.

Follow up or rebuttal reports are often necessary because of the back and forth that goes on between attorneys and experts. I have been involved in larger cases when the plaintiff's attorney hired two or even three experts, and the defense hired one or two experts, all of whom had expertise regarding hazards and falls. Each expert reviewed and reacted to each of the other's reports. Fine points and details got dissected and scrutinized by both sides over and over again. I often agree with some points by other experts, but not with other points. If the case goes to trial, sometimes the small differences in opinion can drive a jury crazy. Hence the term, the battle of the experts.

Don't Fake It!

Whatever you do, do not fake a fall or try to get compensation for a previous injury. Your previous medical record is discoverable, and nowadays security cameras are everywhere. I have seen two cases of fraud in 40 years, and both times plaintiffs faked falls with false claims on what turned out to be old injuries. Both individuals were exposed and were fortunate not to go to prison. One of the plaintiffs dropped his case after security tapes surfaced showing that he clearly staged the falling event, and the other case was dropped after the plaintiff's story and medical records were carefully scrutinized.

Surveillance videos can work for you or against you. Security cameras are commonplace in public spaces and commercial buildings. In a recent case I reviewed the recorded statement of the plaintiff and also examined the surveillance video that showed her tripping and falling. I noted two major discrepancies between what she said happened in her recorded statement and what I saw in the video and the photos taken after she fell. She said the flooring material was concrete on both sides of the edge strip where she tripped, but photos clearly showed that there were two different materials, wood on one side of the tripping hazard, and concrete on the other side. She also said she was carrying bags that blocked her view, but the video showed that she was not carrying anything when she tripped and fell. Neither of these facts changed my opinion that there was an unsafe condition because the vertical change in elevation where she tripped and fell was 0.5in. (12.7mm) high, was not beveled, and it was clearly a tripping hazard that did not comply with ADA Standards or industry standards.

The lesson here is obvious, always tell the truth, the whole truth, and nothing but the truth. Do not embellish the truth. If you do not remember some of the details, just say you do not remember, don't try to fill in the blanks.

There is research that shows that memories of events are not always reliable. It is a human tendency to fill in details where they are missing, and sometimes people 'rewrite' in small ways what happened in the past. Each time someone recalls an event, their memory of that event might change slightly. Therefore, it is important to give a recorded statement as soon after the falling event as possible, and to be as accurate and truthful about the event as you can.

Who Is Really at Fault?
Based on my experience, almost all falls involve both human inattention or carelessness and physical/environmental factors. People expect their environment to be predictable and to follow design and construction standards. But when things are just a little bit off, they often go unnoticed and falls result. For example, everyone expects to encounter a consistent riser height and a consistent tread length in public stairways in newly constructed buildings. If those dimensions are off, even by as little as 0.5in. (12.7mm), the deviation can be enough to cause a trip when going up or down the stairway.

Since our eyes do not take photographs of what we see, we rely on our memory for a record of what occurred. But after someone falls they have a tendency to recall the event in a way that disproportionally blames others and to blame imperfections in the environment. Although most falls do involve environmental issues and/or hazards, people who fall frequently have the tendency to remember their falling event in a favorable way. This is known as "hindsight bias." In other words, it is often difficult for people who fall to accurately recall their falling event accurately and to recognize their own behavior or inattention and the role they may have played.

Takeaways
I woulda paid attention - if only you had mentioned
The act of falling is fast, but recovering from a fall can be a long and arduous process. It is important for a person who falls to recognize their own degree of negligence before filing a lawsuit. After hiring an attorney and filing a lawsuit, it is often best to try to settle the matter through negotiations rather than going to trial. Reasonable agreements can often be reached when attorneys on both sides agree that the defense is more than 50% responsible, and a costly trial can be avoided. If the dispute cannot be settled, a jury will determine who is more negligent, the plaintiff or the defense. When taking a case to trial it is important to be realistic and remember that the legal system is not perfect, and outcomes are unpredictable.

Chapter 11

Reducing Your Risk and Taking Responsibility: Strategies That Work

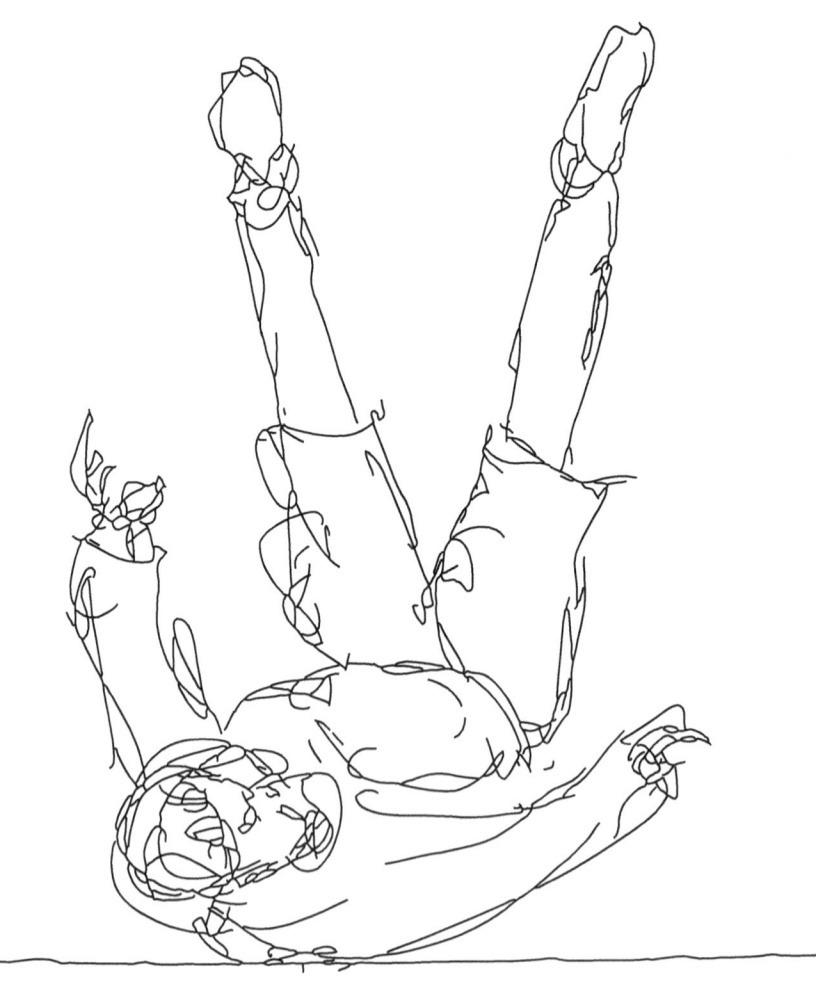

Fear of Falling

We have probably all feared falling from high places when we were younger, as it is a natural part of growing up. When I was a youth I had a very intense fear of falling, and throughout my teenage years I had repeating dreams when I fell (or almost fell) off cliffs, mountain paths, and other high places. I remember being petrified while walking on high bridges and looking down. My heart would race, and I would blush and break out in a sweat whenever I encountered unusual heights. When I was fifteen I decided it was time to try and address my fear, so while I was on a camping trip I chose to climb to the top of Half Dome in Yosemite National Park. I am sure my four companions did not realize or care about my anxiety, but I remember trembling when we started up the granite domed surface. Somehow I made it to the top and back down to the valley below without falling. That trip represented a turning point for me, but I still feel my heart race when I climb to the top of a church or state capitol dome or climb up a tree to get on a zip line.

Maybe having a healthy fear of falling has kept me alive throughout my National Park visits, but I seem to have no fear of falling while walking down the sidewalk. I probably would have fallen less often in my life if

I had at least a little bit of that healthy fear of falling while walking or riding a bicycle.

During the past week four friends of mine fell. A fellow professor slipped and fell on a textured detectable warning surface on a curb ramp as she walked to her car after work. Her face hit the pavement and she suffered facial injuries and serious bruising that will take several months to heal. She told me afterwards that she was being extremely careful when she walked down the curb ramp because she thought it might be slippery, but she fell anyway. Another professor was walking across the parking lot when she encountered a small section of black ice (ice that is hidden, transparent, and/or difficult to see) and her feet went out from under her. She fell backwards, hit her head, and is currently recovering from a concussion.

Then my neighbor fell down the basement stairway in her house, despite the fact that she had walked up and down the same stairway hundreds of times before without incident. She had a serious, painful, and very expensive break in her shoulder. The doctor told her she would have to wait two weeks for the swelling to go down before he could operate and set the break. Surgeons will insert a plate and a pin, and she is expected to recuperate slowly over the next several months.

Another friend put on a new pair of boots and was walking down the hallway in her apartment building when the toe section of one boot got hung up on the carpeting. Although the carpeting was new and securely attached, when the boot caught on the carpet, it was enough to send her flying. She broke her hip, is currently recovering from surgery, and will need to use a walker from this day forward. She said later that it was the first time she had worn her new boots. They had a rubberized toe that she was just getting used to, and she apparently dragged her foot.

All four friends were unfortunate to have suffered falls and injuries, but they were also fortunate that their injuries were not worse, and all of them are on the road to recovery.

Anywhere and Everywhere

Falls are an epidemic in the USA and throughout the world, and the extent of the problem should not be underestimated. You can fall and get injured at any age or any stage of life. Falls happen to all of us and they are inevitable, especially for young children and older adults. One third of older adults fall each year, and after they fall their chances of falling again increase significantly.

Throughout this book I have described hazards in the environment and a wide variety of missteps including slips, trips, airsteps, over-steps, under-steps, and unstable footing that resulted in falls. The point is that there are many ways to fall. Walking is a complex task that requires postural control and balance as you constantly shift your body weight through space. You can think of normal walking as almost falling with each and every step or being barely under control of staying upright. To maintain a smooth gait, you need to coordinate your various body parts to maintain balance while continuously repositioning your center of gravity. Most of the time you do this without thinking about it, but it does not take much to lose your balance. Various things can throw you off, including a sore back, the side effects of medications, or irregularities in the built environment such as small changes in the walking surface.

You may think that what you have been reading to this point is all just 'common sense'. But ask yourself if it is really common sense, then why isn't it very common? One way to look at it is that it is only common sense after you realize what caused you to fall. Remember that most falls don't have to happen, and the vast majority of falls are preventable by changing human behavior. Eliminate the human error and you will reduce your chances of falling to a minimum. Most falls also involve environmental factors that often would be easy and inexpensive to eliminate, especially those in your own home where most falls occur.

Stacking the Odds

A tripping hazard might be present for a long time before you are just unlucky enough to happen to catch the toe of your shoe on it. You may have walked across it dozens of times without incident. You may have successfully negotiated a short step at the bottom of a stairway for years before falling, but all it takes is one time and the result can be disastrous.

Learn to expect falling hazards to be present when you are walking on sidewalks and going in and out of buildings, because falling hazards are commonplace. You can stack the odds in your favor by staying vigilant, maintaining proper lookout, having good footwear, proceeding at a safe speed, staying aware of your surroundings, and not texting or distracting yourself while walking.

Learning How to Fall

I have noticed that people who have been drinking alcohol are often very relaxed and when they fall their bodies are loose. They typically do not fight or resist their falls, and often fall without serious injury. However, drinking too much alcohol can put you at great peril, and can result in a very bad or deadly fall. But if you learn to relax and stay loose when you start to fall you will be less prone to injury. Be mentally prepared to fall because eventually "we all fall down."

Once you have lost your balance and have no chance of recovery, stay relaxed and accept the fact that you are falling. If you panic, it can lead to poor body control. Don't fall with outstretched arms and hands because it will increase your chances of breaking your hands, wrists, arms and shoulders. If you hit hard on your side, you might break your hip. Instead keep your hands tucked in close to your body and your arms and legs loose and bent at the elbows and knees. Reduce the impact by tucking and rolling as you fall to spread out the impact, always protect your head, and don't allow your head to hit hard surfaces.

There are many good resources for learning how to fall safely. All of them advise to always protect your head. This may involve lowering your head, bringing your bent arms up over your head, and falling on another part of your body to avoid hitting your head. If you turn as you fall, you may be able to avoid more serious injuries than you might get from a straight forward, or straight backwards, fall.

If you can do it safely, keep rolling to reduce the impact. Experts advise that you try to avoid landing directly on your hip. Instead try to land on the meaty part of your body where bones have better protection. If you fall forward, tuck and roll, and don't try to abruptly stop yourself. If you fall backwards, tuck your chin so the back of your head does not hit the surface you're falling on.

The key is to mentally program yourself in advance because, when you fall, you will not have time to think about it. Run through it in your mind in advance over and over again, so when it happens you hopefully will not get hurt.

Getting Training

Wouldn't it be great if we were all taught how to fall? If we were all trained to fall when we were young, we would fall less often and have fewer injuries from falls throughout our life span. Requiring fall training in high school would benefit all of society. We require driver's education, so why don't we require fall training? I admire the way soccer and football players know how to fall. Have you ever noticed the way they control their bodies and the way they roll? An interesting study would be to research retired soccer and football players to determine if they have fewer falls and/or fewer injuries from falls than the rest of the population.

I guess in a way I have had my fall training by falling hundreds of times throughout my life. Although I experienced most of those falls before the age of fifty, now that I am seventy-five, or halfway to my goal, I don't really want to fall any more, unless of course I roll it out without being injured.

It is important to practice safe falling with professional help, such as highly skilled physical education teachers, physical therapists, coaches, and personal trainers who can help you learn and practice safe falling techniques in gyms that are equipped with good lighting and heavy padding on the floor. When you practice falling, always be aware of where your head is and protect it as you fall. Practice falling forward while bending your neck forward and tucking in your chin. Practice falling on your side. Practice the tuck and roll while not using your hands and arms to break your fall. Practice falling backwards while staying aware of where your head is, so it does not hit the surface.

Staying Fit

Develop a realistic physical fitness and exercise routine. As we age, it is very important to keep up with our conditioning and to maintain muscle strength and bone density, coordination, and balance. People who are more active are less likely to fall and less likely to sustain serious injury when they do fall. Walking, bicycling, swimming, and other activities help you to maintain your balance and are good for your muscles, bones, and circulatory and respiratory systems. Water exercises increase strength and improve flexibility and are good for your heart and circulatory system. Stair climbing can improve leg stability and strength but use caution and use handrails if you need to. Tai Chi has been shown to be very beneficial while being less physically demanding than other forms of exercise. Tai Chi involves slow rhythmic movements that improve your confidence, muscle strength, flexibility, and balance. Balance exercises may also be appropriate for five or ten minutes a day. All these activities will make it less likely that you will fall, and less likely that you will be injured when you do fall.

Dizziness can greatly increase your likelihood of falling. If you have dizziness and/or a spinning sensation (vertigo) when you get up out of bed, when you get up out of a chair, or at other times, you may have a common condition known as Benign Paroxysmal Positional Vertigo (BPPV) which results when calcium crystals in one or both ears break loose. Fortunately, the condition can be easily treated by medical professionals who have been trained to use specific repositioning maneuvers. I was being treated for a nerve issue in my lower back when my physical therapist noticed I got dizzy when I stood up after laying on my back. During my session she diagnosed the problem and used the Epley maneuver on me. It was painless, took only a few minutes, and completely eliminated my vertigo and dizziness.

As You Age

As you age you may experience an increased fear of falling, especially if you have fallen recently. Fear of falling often leads to reduced mobility and inactivity, which in turn reduces overall physical fitness. If you allow this to occur, your chances of falling and getting injured from falling increases even more. Staying fit and active is important to prevent the cycle. As you age you may also start to notice some additional tendencies that increase your chances of falling. These include changes in your ability to move about, to maneuver your body, and to maintain your balance. You likely will not see or hear as well as you used to, you likely will need additional light to see well, and you may need more time to gather and process information.

While cats can see well in very dark places, humans cannot. And as you age your eyes will take much longer to adjust to very dark places. It normally takes about thirty minutes for your eyes to adapt to dark conditions, but it can take much longer if you have been in bright sunlight, and the longer you have been in bright sunlight, the longer the adaptation takes. Older eyes also experience a gradual clouding of the lenses as cataracts form, impairing vision by reducing the amount of light that reaches the retina and by scattering light. It is advisable to get cataract surgery as soon as you need to, rather than delaying it. It is also helpful to have an anti-reflective coating on your eyeglasses, and to always keep them clean. (Brody, 2007)

If you have eye diseases or other vision problems you may also be more likely to fall, so it is important for you to have your eyes checked regularly, especially if you wear bifocal or progressive lenses. It is also a good idea to keep a backup pair of glasses with you when you travel, in case your frame breaks or a lens pops out. If you wear dark sunglasses, be aware of changing sky conditions and changing lighting, and be careful when entering dark interior spaces. Avoid using dark sunglasses in normal or subdued lighting. Although it may make you look cool, you may not see as well as you would without them. Hearing loss can also increase your chance of falling by reducing your awareness of your surroundings.

In addition to these normal age-related sensory changes you may acquire additional changes in your vision over time that will make you even more vulnerable to falling. If you develop macular degeneration or glaucoma, you will need to be even more vigilant in watching out for hazards and staying within your limits.

As you age, your reflexes slow and your reaction time makes it harder to regain your balance after shifting your body weight. Various medical conditions also affect your balance and increase your chances of falling. People over eighty-five have the highest risk of falls and are also the fastest growing segment of the population. If you get Parkinson's, Hodgkin's, MS, ALS, or other progressive neurological disorders, you will need to be especially aware of falling hazards. If you have osteoporosis, your bones are more fragile, and falls are very dangerous for you. Medical treatments for these conditions have improved dramatically over the past few years, so make the most of the latest advances. If you have any of these conditions, try to compensate for your increased risk of falling by training yourself to watch out for falling hazards in public places and by eliminating hazards at home.

Many of us find ourselves on multiple prescription medications periodically, or continuously. Unfortunately, many medications, individually and in combination, can make you more susceptible to being light-headed, dizzy, and/or drowsy. Consuming even a little bit of alcohol can make you more vulnerable, and alcohol can also intensify some bad side effects of medications, such as drowsiness or dizziness. Even having allergies or a common head cold can increase your vulnerability.

As you continue to age, you will likely experience changes in your gait and posture. Gait changes often result in slower walking speeds and shorter strides. You may also swing your arms less. These changes typically happen gradually over time but become more noticeable with advancing years and arthritis. However, you can learn to compensate for many of these changes by being aware of them and adjusting to them, and by staying in good physical and mental condition.

If your doctor recommends that you use a cane, a walking stick, or a walker to help you maintain your balance, be extra careful because you may not be able to detect and 'feel' the walking surface in the same way you did before using your walking aide. Using a walker may also change your center of gravity. Be aware of the position of the legs of your walker because they can easily catch on edges or cracks or float off the edges of sidewalks.

If you have conditions that make navigating the environment more difficult, learn and practice ways to compensate. For example, if you have vision loss caused by cataracts, see your ophthalmologist to determine if you are ready for lens replacement surgery. If you are not to the point where surgery is appropriate, compensate for your vision loss by walking slower, being more cautious, and using handrails. If you have hearing loss, see an audiologist and get fitted with hearing aids and then use them rather than letting them sit in a dresser drawer. If you have a mobility problem, make the appropriate changes in your behavior. If you have multiple issues, use multiple strategies to compensate and reduce your chances of falling.

Dogs and Cats

In the USA emergency room visits from falls caused by dogs and cats total more than 86,000 each year. About two thirds of the falls associated with cats and one third of the falls associated with dogs are caused by falling over them. More than 20% of falls associated with dogs are caused by the person being pushed or pulled by a dog. Falling over a pet item, like a toy or food bowl, accounted for almost 9% of fall injuries (cdc.gov).

People need to be especially careful when walking dogs on leashes. Dogs can suddenly lunge at other dogs or animals and forcefully pull on the leash. Retractable leashes can make the problem worse because dogs can get a running start before causing an even bigger jolt forward. Older people who have limited strength and slower reaction time need to be especially careful with large dogs.

While deaths are rare from pet related falls, they do happen. Susie Jacobson, a 62-year-old woman who worked out regularly and trained six days a week was walking her 80 pound (36.3 kilos) golden retriever when her dog unexpectedly lunged toward another dog. She fell and hit her head on the sidewalk. After she fell she was alone at home where she later died from her head injury (Zorn, 2019).

Good obedience training for dogs will help, but it is almost impossible to prevent dogs from behaving 100% of the time like dogs naturally want to behave, and good luck trying obedience training with a cat!

Minimizing Distractions
Distractions make it difficult to pay attention to hazards, and you typically experience many visual and auditory distractions while walking and while ascending and descending a stairway. Distractions are a major cause, or contributing cause, of a very high percentage of falls. Pay attention to the task of walking and don't let distractions throw you off. When you sense you are being distracted, slow down or stop and refocus your attention on what is ahead.

Sometimes the distraction is the result of your own actions. In fact, we all distract ourselves while walking. For example, we have all rushed, thought about other things, not paid attention to our walking, and become less consciously aware of our surroundings. We have all carried things such as purses, briefcases, coffee mugs, children or pets, laundry baskets, clothes, and boxes. We have all talked to others, laughed, or looked at our watches while walking. However, distractions have increased dramatically now that we have smart phones that allow us to text, read, surf the internet, listen to music, or watch a video while walking. But just because you can do these things doesn't mean it is a good idea. We may think it is 'not a big deal' because we have gotten away with it before. But keep in mind, research shows that we don't multitask very well, if at all. Instead we actually switch our attention back and forth between tasks.

Other distractions caused by your surroundings also pull your visual and auditory attention away from your most important task at hand, walking. Being aware of this is especially important when you are on a stairway. There are often activities going on in other spaces near a stairway such as people talking or moving about. There are often pictures on the wall, changing lighting conditions, reflections and shadows. Stair coverings can also be distracting, especially when they are multicolored and patterned. Since you are not able to eliminate these types of distractions when you are in public places, you must learn to minimize your increased risk of falling by remembering that your primary responsibility is to yourself to successfully navigate the stairway without incident. Don't make the situation worse by adding unnecessary distractions of your own. We often need to carry things and talk to others. We don't need to live in cocoons; we just need to be aware and cautious.

Taking Risks

No situation is ever totally risk free. Think of what you experienced when you tried to avoid getting the Covid-19 virus. It was almost impossible to avoid risk entirely. You knew you could reduce your risk substantially by wearing a mask, not getting close to people, staying outdoors, and avoiding indoor places that were crowded with people. The goal was to minimize your risk, but not necessarily to eliminate it entirely. If you went to the doctor's office, or the pharmacy or the grocery store you assumed some level of risk. But some risk can also be a good thing. We have learned that limited exposure to the virus may be beneficial for some people because it helps us build up our immunity. If we had not played in the dirt as children we would have weaker immunity.

Every time you get up and walk anywhere you are taking some risk, but that does not mean you should never walk again. If I had not stumbled and fallen many times in my life, I believe I would be at greater risk of falling and being injured during a fall.

When I was very young I broke my arm riding a tricycle and then broke the same arm again a few years later riding my bicycle. Both times I was going too fast. My brother learned how to ride his bike backwards while sitting on his handlebars. He did it on many occasions until one day he lost his balance, fell and broke his arm. My cousin walked backwards while talking to me, but when he walked into a bush he fell backwards over the bush and broke his wrist. All of these falling incidents can be explained by risky and careless adolescent behavior. When we are young we don't think about blaming someone else for what we do. Instead we accept that "It was my fault," and it usually was.

As adults we tend to take fewer risks when it comes to careless behaviors. But as adults, and especially as older adults, a small mistake or oversight can have big consequences. Imagine tripping on a crack that is only 0.75in. (19.1mm) high and breaking both shoulders because you extended your arms out in front of you when you fell. Imagine not seeing a step down in front of you, taking an airstep, and ending up with a serious injury. Imagine slipping on a wet floor and falling on your elbow. These things happen to people who don't think of themselves as being careless. If you recognize that these events might happen to you, you are more likely to be observant and spot hazards, thus making it less likely that you will fall.

If you leave an extension cord on the floor where you walk, you are taking a risk that you might trip on it. You knowingly take the risk. It is your choice, your decision, and your risk. You know what is best, but you still take the risk. You are thinking to yourself, "I know it is there so I will be careful and step over it." But if you trip and fall, you will have no one to blame but yourself. However, if a friend or family member trips and falls, you will have to live with the fact that you could have eliminated the hazard but chose not to.

You also take a risk walking down a stairway in a public building when the bottom stair riser is shorter than the rest of the risers in the stairway. If you know it is there or even if you don't know it is there, you can compensate and reduce your risk of falling by holding onto the handrail.

Minimizing Risk

All of us take risks all the time, but there seems to be a prevailing attitude that "it won't happen to me." You might have been up and down a stairway hundreds of times, causing you to minimize the risk in your mind. You feel safe because you have done it so many times before, so you are not fully aware of the risk you are taking. But the unsafe condition is still there waiting for you. The risk is still there, even though you did not fall before. And the consequences of falling down a stairway can be significant. If you are lucky enough not to hit your head or break your bones, you will likely have bruises, sprains, and trauma to deal with. Why is it that so many people do not use handrails most of the time? Maybe it is because they are not aware of the risk, or maybe they think the risk is miniscule. However, if you consistently use handrails, you will reduce your risk of falling. Stop and consider the many ways we place ourselves at risk of falling and then develop strategies to minimize those risks.

Taking Control and Responsibility

We live in a world where we are desperately trying to keep things under control all the time. None of us want to lose control of our bodies or body parts, like bladders and hair. We try to control what we wear, our smiles, and our posture. We even try to hold back our sweat, so it does not show.

With regards to falling we try not to fall, we try not to get hurt when we do fall, and not to admit falling to anyone except spouses after we fall, unless of course we are seen falling. In that case we either laugh at ourselves or cry out for help.

I had a vision recently of wearing a balloon outfit where I could put on a series of Velcro strapped bubble wrapped belts around my hips, shoulders, elbows, knees, ankles, and head so I could enjoy falling and bouncing around without getting hurt.

If each of us took more responsibility for our own actions, the number of falls would be greatly reduced. Why is the concept of 'personal responsibility' so difficult to instill in our society? By observing falling hazards and walking around or over them you are being responsible to yourself. Sometimes it means taking more time, sometimes it means taking a longer route, sometimes it means taking short baby steps, and sometimes it means using walking aides or depending on others for help. Whatever it calls for, safe behavior starts with being in the present, recognizing your responsibility to observe, and then acting appropriately for the circumstances.

Our lack of responsibility is partly due to the fast-paced lives we live, where distractions are everywhere and multi-tasking behavior, which is dominated by our digital culture, is viewed as desirable. We all want to make every minute count to the fullest extent possible, but we should not do so at the expense of our own safety.

When I was a teenager, the car I was driving was rear-ended and although I was not seriously injured, I had a sore neck for many weeks. The auto insurance company wanted me to settle and even suggested that I get medical attention and physical therapy. I said I just wanted to wait and make sure that the whiplash I experienced in my car without headrests did not result in a long term problem. Every few weeks the insurance company called me and asked me if I was ready to close the case. Each time they called I said I did not want a settlement, I just wanted to make sure I was ok. After about three months I felt better and notified the insurance company that I was ready to sign off. I could not believe it when I received a check in the mail for one hundred dollars with a note thanking me for my cooperation. That was a lot of money for me to receive unexpectedly at the time. My goal was not to get a windfall, it was to make sure I was okay before agreeing to close the file.

There is one more important point I need to bring up about my rear-end accident. The driver that drove into me said the brake lights on my car were not working, and when I tested them I discovered that he was right, they were not working. Therefore I felt at least partially responsible for what had happened.

In today's culture there seems to be a tendency to want to immediately blame others when things go wrong, and to not recognize our own role in what happens. If you take your case to trial, it will ultimately be up to a jury to determine the percentage of fault for both the plaintiff and the defense. However, in most states it is extremely rare for the verdict to be 100% one way or the other. In other words, you are almost always, except in very rare cases, determined to be at least partially responsible for your fall.

You should not completely blame yourself, or completely blame the hazard, or completely blame the people that did not eliminate the hazard. The point is there is plenty of blame, or responsibility, to go around. The more important issue is, what can you do now to take more responsibility in order to reduce your risk?

Times have changed. When people fell years ago, they almost always blamed themselves for their careless behavior, even when there were unsafe conditions present. Let us assume for a minute that it is 'like the old days' again and it is not easy to sue a property owner when you fall, as is still the case in most of the world today. Would this foster safer behavior? Maybe. We need laws and a justice system that fairly compensates those that are wronged, so I do not advocate going back to the past. However, our society would also benefit enormously if each of us, as individuals, would take more responsibility for our own actions.

Think back to how many times you have fallen in your lifetime. You don't remember many of them because you were either very young or you were able to get up again without having injuries. Now think back to the times you remember when you were injured, or at least shaken up enough to remember it. Ask yourself, would those falls have occurred if you had been looking at the path ahead, or if you were wearing better footwear, or if you had not rushed, or if you had not allowed yourself to be distracted? These are all your responsibilities in a world where falling hazards are, and always will be, commonplace.

Your Expectations and Risk Threshold

The challenge is to increase your awareness to the point of keeping you safe, but not to the point of obsession. When you are constantly thinking about falling, you limit your ability to have fun and enjoy life. You need to find your own threshold by training yourself to spot potential hazards and by being aware of your surroundings at all times, but also by not putting unreasonable limits on your desired life activities.

Once you find your own risk threshold, it is a constant challenge to maintain it. As much as I hate to admit it, I sometimes miss important visual cues because I am not paying close enough attention. Recently I walked into a store but was not aware of the fact that I had actually stepped up a couple of inches as I walked through the open doorway. So, when I walked out of the store a few minutes later, I took a small airstep because I was not aware of the drop. Thankfully, I have learned to walk cautiously and within my limits most of the time, and I was fortunate to be able to maintain my footing without incident. Even when you happen to miss a visual cue, cautious behavior can prevent a fall.

In addition to your risk threshold, you also have an awareness threshold. Your awareness threshold can be thought of as a certain minimum level of awareness of your surroundings that is needed to stay safe whenever and wherever you move about. Your risk threshold will change over the years as you age and you become more cautious. Your awareness threshold needs to be increased as you age because falls are more likely, and it becomes harder to compensate for missed cues. But if you learn to stay within your safe limit in terms of walking speed and awareness, you can avoid falling. You may stumble a bit from time to time, but you will also have a better chance of recovering your balance if you stay aware, stay fit, and stay within your own appropriate speed limit.

It is helpful to think about the role our own 'expectations' play in falls. For example, we have come to expect that all of the risers in a typical stairway will be the same height. This expectation is based on our previous experiences with stairways, and we have no reason to expect otherwise. Since both the ADA Standards and the International Building Code (IBC) prohibit deviations in riser height to be more than 0.38in. (9.0mm), most stairways actually conform to this requirement. However, some stairways either were not built to meet the standard, or flooring materials added at the top of the stairway increased the top riser height.

So when we walk down a stairway that we are unfamiliar with, where the top riser is an inch or more higher than the other risers in the stairway, we are not expecting to encounter an unusually high step. To make it worse, it is more difficult to observe the deviation when we are descending the stairway because we don't have the same visual cues we have when walking up the stairway. This is because we do not see the riser when we are descending the stairway, and because the surfaces of the stair treads tend to blend together. So unless we are expecting the deviation, we may not notice it.

Another example of where expectations can be a factor is a curb ramp. The ADA Standards have specific requirements regarding curb ramp design, slopes, and dimensions and we have come to expect curb ramps we encounter to be at least reasonably close to meeting those design standards. So when we unexpectedly encounter an unusually steep curb ramp that does not conform to the standards we are accustomed to, it can throw off our footing and our balance. And in a similar way to the stairway example, it may be difficult to observe that the curb ramp is unusually steep before we encounter it because it is hard to tell how steep sloped surfaces really are.

Natasha Barkley walked out of a restaurant on her way to a car that was waiting for her in a circular drive/drop off area that served several businesses and a hotel. When she stepped onto what looked to her like a flat concrete strip, she experienced unstable footing, twisted her foot and fell sideways, breaking her ankle in the process. When I inspected the location where she fell, I determined that the concrete strip was not actually flat. Instead there was a non-standard sloped curb that separated a patterned tile sidewalk and the brick paved circular drive/drop off area. The curb had a standard curb profile in the center section of the circular drive where the hotel entrance was, but it gradually smoothed down to become an almost flat strip of concrete. The concrete transition strip served as a visual separation between the tiled sidewalk and the brick street, but it was difficult to detect the sloped surface in the location where Natasha fell that was in between the section with the standard curb profile and the flat section at the other end. It looked flat to Natasha when she stepped on it.

The designer had created an attractive setting with regards to paving materials, but the concrete dividing strip that started out as a standard curb at one end and gradually flattened out was a hazard, especially where there were unfamiliar non-standard slopes that were difficult to recognize.

The problem is that people do not recognize that there is a sloped surface, or if they do, they do not understand the severity of the slope that they are about to step on. Then they have difficulty getting secure footing, especially when approaching from an angle. Even when people recognize the unusual configuration, they may misjudge the degree of slope when they step onto it.

When we walk on cobblestone we expect uneven surfaces and when we climb stairs on ancient buildings and sites we expect the stairs will be irregular. As a result, we are more careful when we navigate them. But when we are walking up or down a stairway in a modern building we expect the stairs to be dimensionally consistent. Therefore, when a stairway in a new building is just a little bit out of compliance with standards, it can be very hazardous because we have learned to expect the treads and risers within a stairway to be dimensionally consistent. So, when they are just a little bit off, even as little as 0.5in. (12.7mm), we may not notice the difference and may miss-step as a result.

The Benefits of a Hazardous Environment

Would we all be safer and less at risk of falling if our environment was not as safe? It might sound counter intuitive, but this may be at least partially true. I recall staying at a bed and breakfast in England a few years ago where our room was on the second floor in a centuries old house. The only way to get to our room was to walk up a very odd and steep curved stairway that had a wall around it but no handrails. The individual stair treads were not uniform in terms of profile or dimension, and the stairway would definitely not comply with modern building codes. I remember when I first walked up the stairway I thought to myself, "This stairway is very unsafe." However, both my wife and I found ourselves being extremely careful every time we went up or down the stairway. I soon realized that because the stairway was so unusual and different from the stairways we normally experience, the non-compliant stairway was, in a way, actually safer because it forced us to be extremely cautious.

Neighborhoods in San Francisco and other cities throughout the world have extremely steep streets and sidewalks with slopes ranging between 20 and 30%. Those sidewalks far exceed the maximum 8.3% slopes for ramps permitted by the ADA Standards, making them very difficult or impossible for wheelchair users and other people with disabilities to safely navigate. However, residents who live in those neighborhoods routinely walk up and down very steep slopes without incident. They have learned to adjust their walking to navigate the steep slopes without falling. But just because steep sidewalks exist does not mean that they are safe for everyone. Steep sidewalks that are safely navigated by some people are not safely negotiated by other people, such as people with mobility or balance problems.

Standards and Codes Do Not Guarantee Your Safety

One of the problems with standards and codes is that they don't always prescribe the best way to design or build. Instead, they represent minimum standards. For example, the ADA Standards provide minimum dimensions for turning wheeled mobility devices, but the minimum dimensions were based on maneuvering a standard wheelchair and today there are more electric scooters than wheelchairs. Many users have difficulty maneuvering through spaces that are designed and constructed to meet minimum wheelchair requirements. In *Access for Everyone* I provide hundreds of recommendations that go beyond minimum requirements. However, the continuing development of these recommendations is a never-ending process, so the reader is encouraged to always think beyond minimums (see *Access for Everyone* for specific recommendations).

When it comes to safety issues related to falls, neither the building code nor the ADA Standards include many needed and useful recommendations. For example, contrasting edge strips on stair treads have been known to increase safety and reduce the number of falls for more than 40 years, but this was only recently mentioned in some new codes and is still not in the ADA Standards. Another example is that the color of handrails should contrast the color of walls they are mounted on, to make them easier to see.

Seeing and Observing Falling Hazards

There is a big difference between seeing and observing. Observation is a skill we can learn to improve that involves not just seeing but paying attention. We have allowed our minds to wander much of the time, even though we were not always aware of doing it. We all tend to filter out many things we see as we walk, so we must make identifying hazards a priority in order to properly observe them. If we don't think of them as a priority, then our minds will not have sharp observation skills for recognizing hazards.

It is important for us to increase our awareness of our physical surroundings, including surface conditions and irregularities, slopes, colors, lighting, shadows, and contrast. We can learn to observe hazards with conscious awareness rather than just seeing them. We need to pay attention to the walking surface and what we see one or two steps in front of us, and to watch out for surfaces that blend together visually where there might be small changes in elevation. Small changes in surfaces can be hazardous because we are less likely to see them, and a trip on a height difference of only 0.25in. (6.4mm) can lead to serious injury.

We need to learn to observe stairs carefully before we walk up or down on them to see if the top riser or the bottom riser are a different height than those in the rest of the stairway. We should be able to discern if the stairs are sloped to one side, if they are uneven with inconsistent tread and riser sizes, if the handrails look sturdy, if the handrails are located where we need them, and if they are easy to grasp. If we don't see it ahead of time, an increased step height of as little as 1.5in. (38.1mm) or a step down onto a sloped surface can result in an airstep and a broken hip.

Learning to observe better requires conscious thought and self-discipline to pay attention where necessary. Our eyes have a narrow field of vision in sharp focus while most of what we see at any given moment is through our peripheral vision. But peripheral vision is also blurry vision, so our eyes dart around constantly to pick up important information. When we become overly familiar with our environment we have a tendency to observe less and may not notice small changes that have occurred, like a new tripping hazard where a section of a sidewalk has settled. Another problem with familiarity is that we become over confident, and that can lead to less accurate observations, making us more susceptible to hazards.

Better observations lead to better awareness, better awareness leads to better behavior, and better behavior leads to fewer falls, injuries, and lawsuits. While walking we should visually scan at least five to ten feet ahead to detect falling hazards. If you see something that looks suspicious like a heaved section of concrete, or a severe cross-slope, or a deviation in the surface, observe it carefully as you get closer and then step over it or walk around it. If we know a hazard is in front of us, we can avoid falling. If we don't know it is there, we increase our chances of falling.

We have all heard the following statement over and over again: "Human beings only use ten percent of their brains." This statement is both untrue and very misleading. Research has proven that we use almost our entire brain much of the time, and that information overload can lead to unsafe behavior (Boyd, 2008). Overscheduling, multitasking, and mobile communication devices all contribute to information bombardment. Staying safe requires us to selectively direct our attention to deal with information overload. There are many reasons why people don't recognize hazards, but most of the time it is a case of not observing them.

All of us have multiple falling hazards in and around our own homes that we have learned to walk around, and most of the time we know where they are and are able to avoid them. We also know that we should eliminate them, but until we do, at least we know where they are. However, a fall occurs suddenly and can happen at any time, even when you have known about the presence of a hazard for a long time. All it takes is one mistake, one misstep, one miss-judgement, one distraction, and you can trip on a throw rug or an extension cord or a shoe you left on the floor. Think of them as hazards waiting for you to find them, instead of obstacles that you can walk over or around.

Don't Rely on Warnings

A warning can help alert people so they detect a hazard they might not otherwise observe. I am using the term 'detect' to mean a 'conscious awareness'. Without a conscious awareness it is easy to miss a hazard. A warning can be effective in catching our attention, but not for everyone or in every situation.

If you know you have a tripping hazard on your sidewalk, you can paint the vertical and horizontal edges of the elevation change with a bright color paint until you have time to have someone fix it. Remember this does not correct the unsafe condition, it only warns people about it. Painted warnings fade or get covered with snow and can be missed in poor weather conditions or poor lighting or crowded conditions that limit or negate their effectiveness. Someone may not see a painted warning at night or when they are walking with a group of people. Also, a painted warning may not be effective at alerting a person who has limited vision and will be completely ineffective as a warning to most blind people.

There are also problems with warning cones and folding signs that are placed over or near spill hazards or wet floors in stores. Cones and portable folding signs do not define the limits of a spill if it is difficult to see, and spills tend to spread. Cones and folding signs can also be easily moved, where at least the painted edge of a tripping hazard can't be moved. Another problem with safety cones and folding warning signs is that we get used to them being everywhere, so we learn to ignore them. Most of the time when I see them, the floor is already dry. Store employees need to remove them as soon as the area is dry, not an hour or two later. Therefore a warning can be helpful in some circumstances but remember that a warning does not correct an unsafe condition.

Multi-Tasking While Walking and Sensory Overload

In today's hyper-active world we think we can do multiple things at the same time. However, research has shown that our ability to multitask is greatly overrated because we are actually switching back and forth between activities rather than 'multi-tasking'.

Multi-tasking is different than carrying on an activity while one of them is almost automatic. For example, we can walk and talk to someone next to us at the same time because walking has become automatic and does not require conscious thought most of the time. We can unload the dishwasher or fold clothes while we listen to the news on the radio or television because we are not consciously thinking about what we are doing with our hands. But when we try to find a phone number on our phone while we are driving, it requires us to take our attention away from the task of driving. In this case we may think we are multi-tasking, but we are actually switching our attention back and forth between activities, and a two-second distraction while driving can result in driving over the lane line, or worse.

Although walking is second nature for most of us most of the time, it can be a costly mistake to lower our level of awareness. When college campus buildings have signs posted in stairways warning students not to text while walking on a stairway, we know that our society has a problem with multi-tasking. In my opinion it is not good practice to post anything in a stairway because reading a sign can itself be an unsafe distraction.

In our modern world we experience sensory overload daily. We squeeze into crowded noisy sports bars or restaurants that have multiple flat screen televisions blaring various games at us, with each one demanding our attention. Single steps, high door thresholds, and changing floor materials become more hazardous if you don't see them because you are preoccupied processing extra information. The last thing you are thinking about is slipping or tripping. You can minimize the sensory overload by choosing a smaller and quieter restaurant or by eating during times when they are less crowded, or by eating at home.

Another example is a crowded airport where you are bombarded with endless repeating recorded messages, people talking, music playing, lights glaring, reflections on highly polished floors, and hard to read flight information displays and confusing signs. All of this is happening while your ears are ringing from your last flight and you are trying to get the feeling back in your legs again after sitting too long. Simultaneously, you are trying to find the nearest restroom, determine how long it will take to get to the next gate, and whether or not you should grab something to eat or start running. But be aware that running may not be safe and sensory overload can increase your chances of falling because you are more likely to miss important visual cues. You can minimize the impact of sensory overload in the airport by traveling on Saturday, staying well rested, and wearing noise-cancelling headphones on noisy planes, or better yet, take the train.

Lighting

Low lighting is frequently a contributing factor to falls. Learn to stop in your tracks, when it is safe to do so, to let your eyes adjust to dark areas. The classic example of this is when you walk into a dark interior space on a bright sunny day. You experience temporary blindness until your eyes adjust, so wait inside the front door for a few minutes before going further. Then go slow and use extra caution until your eyes adjust to the low lighting. Know your own limits and avoid being heroic by trying to keep up with others. Tell them to go ahead or ask them to slow down.

Lighting levels at dusk, when the sun is setting, can vary tremendously with changing weather conditions and changing seasons. Low lighting situations in public areas are a common problem in many cities, towns, and rural communities. Go slow and avoid venturing into areas where it is too dark to see tripping and falling hazards.

Be aware of artificial lighting systems that can make colors appear to shift into different colors and can affect both contrast level and depth perception. Depressions in parking lots, tripping hazards, and slopes on sidewalks can be more difficult to see under artificial lighting. Go slower to compensate.

Footwear

Make sure to have good slip resistant footwear that fits properly. Many people fall while wearing loose fitting flip-flops or poorly fitting or worn-out shoes with smooth soles. We would all benefit from wearing different shoes with different types of soles for various weather conditions. A common problem is smooth bottoms on footwear due to excessive wear which can substantially reduce slip resistance. Ask yourself, is it worth it to keep those unsafe worn-out shoes just because they are comfortable?

Being Present

I first heard the term "be here now" in a woodshop training class while learning how to use power tools because it is of utmost importance to be in the present moment and not to be thinking about the past or dreaming about the future. It makes perfect sense, don't allow yourself to think about something else while using a power saw. You can cut your finger off in a split second. One of the best carpenters I know is missing the end of a finger because he sawed it off. "Be here now" really makes sense in the woodshop.

Have you ever been driving your car while trying to tune your radio or adjusting your mirror, or looking at a map on the screen when you suddenly realize you have taken your eyes off the road and your attention away from the responsibility of driving for more than a few seconds? I have.

When I was in high school, all students were required to take driver's education. One thing my teacher said back then, before the days of seat belts and air bags, that stuck with me all these years is: "If you are driving along the road and suddenly realize that you have not been thinking about your driving for the last few moments, then you should not be driving." Taking your attention away from your driving for just a few seconds can cost you your life.

The same can be said for walking over uneven surfaces or on stairways. One missed visual cue may be all it takes for you to miss a step and, once you start to fall, you fall very fast. It is a good idea to be present in the moment and to remember the phrase "be here now" wherever you go.

Spotting Hazards
Trippers

Trippers are very common in colder climates when sections of concrete sidewalks heave or drop due to freeze-thaw cycles. Trippers are also common at doorways that have high thresholds. And they are common between parking lot surfaces and sidewalks, between curbs and sidewalks, at curb ramps, between brick and concrete surfaces, where tree roots have cracked sidewalks, near manhole covers, and where cracks occur anywhere in the walking surface. When you see bright colored tape or paint on a tripper, chances are that someone else has already fallen there.

Train yourself to observe small elevation changes or 'trippers' in walkways and routes. This starts by watching out for all cracks, control joints, and construction joints in all sidewalks and exterior walking surfaces. Control joints are those scored lines perpendicular to the direction of travel that typically appear at 5ft. (1.52m) intervals in the sidewalks. They are there to encourage the inevitable cracks to occur there rather than in random places throughout the sidewalk.

Construction joints are used to separate different concrete pours to allow for expansion and contraction. They are less frequent than control joints, but they often result in tripping hazards when freeze-thaw cycles occur or when settling or heaving occurs. When cracks in concrete occur along control joints, they are often followed by movement up or down in the adjacent sections of concrete. When changes in height are less than 0.25in. (6.4mm) they are "within standard" but can still be a tripping hazard. The ADA Standards require vertical changes that are over 0.25in. (6.4mm) but less than 0.5in. (12.7mm) to be beveled. However, a vertical change of as little as 0.25in. (6.4mm) can be problematic if you don't see it.

Slippery surfaces

During cold months walking surfaces can turn slippery in a few seconds. Sometimes you have no choice but to walk over a slippery surface, so when you do, go slowly and take small steps or shuffle your feet without lifting them up and maintain your balance by not allowing your feet to get too far away from your body.

Look for locations that may have transparent and therefore hard-to-see 'black ice' or 'clear ice' on the surface, including: low or depressed areas where there are downspouts nearby, and low areas where water can puddle over sections of sidewalk, driveways, or parking lots. You can even slip on ice that is covered with a puddle of water. It can briefly happen on a sunny day when the temperature gets above freezing and snow melt drains over an ice-covered pothole in the shade. This is not something that happens often, but it does happen, proving once again that you must always be on the lookout for the unexpected.

Airsteps

When you approach a step up, it is typically easier to recognize because the riser (the vertical part of the step) appears to be darker because of the lighting, thus calling attention to itself. It is still a tripping hazard, but you are more likely to see it than a step down. When you approach a single step down, it is often difficult to recognize when the surfaces on both sides of the step appear to blend together. But even when a material or color change exists at a step down, you can still misread the two surfaces as one flat surface. Single steps down as small as 1.5in.

(38.1mm) can lead to airsteps and falls. I sometimes refer to airstep hazards as 'hidden hazards' because they are hard to spot, and you don't realize that you are about to step down.

Sloping surfaces at curb ramps and doorways

Sloped surfaces are common at curb ramps and at doorways to older buildings or shops on Main Street where modifications have been made to eliminate single steps by sloping the sidewalk to match up with interior floor surfaces. They also occur where sidewalks cross driveways and where the edges of cracks have been ground down to eliminate trippers. If any of those slopes are excessive, a hazard can result.

Slopes up or down

Sudden, unexpected slopes up or down in the direction of travel (running slopes) can be hazardous if you don't recognize them. Even minor slopes can twist your foot and cause you to lose your footing.

Excessive cross-slopes

Cross-slopes (perpendicular to the direction of travel) in accessible routes that are over 2% are not permitted by the ADA Standards, but I have frequently measured cross-slopes in the range of 4-8%. Excessive cross-slopes are common where overall site grading was not done properly before sidewalks were constructed and where sidewalks settle to one side.

Falls frequently occur on curb ramps and those triangular shaped side-flares on curb ramps. Excessive cross-slopes often result when side-flares are inappropriately warped to match up with existing conditions. A person can lose their footing when stepping on excessive cross-slopes. Cross-slopes are especially hazardous for people who have low vision and people using canes, crutches, walkers, wheelchairs or electric scooters.

Walking on grass

Grass covered slopes can be slippery and treacherous, especially when they are damp or wet. People should be careful when taking shortcuts over turf and grassy areas, and when there may be irregularities and ground squirrel holes that are hard to see. Everyone needs to be especially careful when walking up or down grass covered hillsides. It may be safer to go the longer route to avoid them.

Multi-faceted hazards
Each of the hazardous conditions described above can result in a fall and potentially serious injury. However, many sidewalk and parking lot hazards often have additional problems such as: poor lighting, shadows, visually blending surfaces or poor drainage. Stairways often have inadequate lighting and/or lack of color contrast on the leading edge of stair treads in addition to having uneven stair riser height, sloping treads, handrails that do not have extensions, and/or handrails that are difficult to grasp.

Walking Style
A person does not need to put themselves in harm's way when walking with another person who wants to walk at a faster pace. It may be safer to walk alone. People should also avoid walking too fast for conditions, including: weather conditions, lighting, shadows, surface materials that are too smooth or too rough, and surface irregularities.

Remember that our likelihood of falling varies from day to day and hour to hour. We may be more vulnerable before we have our morning coffee and less vulnerable afterwards. We may get hyped up and careless if we have too much coffee. Medications may also have a negative effect on safe walking. Sitting too long may make us lightheaded or stiff when we stand up. Our eyes may need more time to adjust when coming from a bright area to a dark area. All of us need to listen to our inner voices when they say, "slow down, stay within your limit."

If you observe that a stairway you are about to ascend or descend has safety issues, use extra caution and behave accordingly. Proceed deliberately, grab handrails securely, and take one step at a time.

When we drive a car, we know we are taking a risk, but we accept the risk and don't constantly think about it. But even if we realized how risky driving really was, we would likely drive just as much anyway because it is human nature to venture out, to be independent, and to take control. When we walk on the sidewalk, we assume that we are safe and most of us are not thinking about falling. We assume there is very little risk while walking. However, we don't need to let the act of walking be riskier than it needs to be. Our overall attitude impacts our behavior and cautious behavior can help keep us safe.

Reduce Your Chance of Falling
- Develop good habits
- Program yourself to recognize falling hazards and either negotiate them or avoid them
- Don't assume that hazards ahead of you will grab your attention
- Always be aware of possible environmental hazards such as black ice, changes in route surfaces, uneven stair heights, and loose or missing handrails
- Consciously improve your observation and awareness skills to identify falling hazards
- Train yourself to scan the visual field ahead of you and frequently glance down at walking surfaces
- When you spot a potential tripping hazard, proceed with caution and step over it or around it
- Don't drag your feet too close to the surface, especially over uneven surfaces
- Give yourself enough time to navigate at your own comfortable speed and let others walk ahead if you need to
- Don't walk at a faster speed than you are comfortable with, especially when you are on unfamiliar routes and/or in dark areas
- When running, don't allow your upper body to get too far ahead of your feet which could result in a loss of balance
- Be extra careful to secure good footing when getting in and out of vehicles
- Watch out for loose or worn entrance mats that curl up or have edges that catch the toe of your foot
- Try to keep your hands free to help maintain balance while walking

- When walking a dog with a leash, prepare yourself for sudden forceful pulls
- Leave garage doors in the fully open or fully closed position so they are not head banging and falling hazards

Be prepared to fall
- Mentally prepare yourself to fall, because you probably will fall once in a while
- Practice safe falling on thick floor pads with professional coaches, physical therapists, and trainers
- Maintain, or restore, your overall physical condition with a fitness routine to sustain flexibility and balance

When you fall
- When you fall, don't fight it, stay relaxed and loose, and don't panic
- Keep your arms and legs loose and bent at the elbows and knees
- Protect your head by placing your bent arm next to your head
- If you fall forward, protect your head and roll out the fall, if it is safe to do so, rather than trying to break your fall with your hands and arms
- If you slip and fall backwards, bend your neck and keep your head forward to prevent your head from falling back and hitting the ground
- Try to land on the meatier parts, rather than the bonier parts, of your body
- Be prepared to let go of things you are carrying

Don't fall for distractions
- Focus your primary attention on walking and avoid unnecessary distractions, such as looking at your phone
- Don't let unavoidable distractions modify your walking behavior
- Stop in you tracks when you need to, but only when it is safe to do so

Learn how to carry things
- Use a shoulder bag, fanny pack or backpack to keep your hands free
- Be careful when carrying things, especially when your arms are not free to move to help you maintain your balance
- Don't block your view with items you are carrying
- Don't carry too many items at a time or items that are too large or too heavy
- Make more trips with fewer items instead of carrying large loads

Adjust to changing lighting and impaired vision
- Give your eyes enough time to adjust to changing lighting, especially when walking from a bright exterior to a dark interior
- Be aware of artificial lighting that can change the appearance of surfaces and reduce your vision
- Watch out for shadow patterns that camouflage the edges of steps and irregularities in sidewalks
- Be aware of changing weather and sky conditions that reduce your vision
- Don't wear extremely dark sunglasses in moderate lighting conditions when it might impair your vision

Wear safe clothing and footwear
- Wear slacks that fit properly, and not slacks that are too long and might cause you to trip over them
- Use appropriate footwear with the proper slip resistance for the given weather conditions (dry, wet, snow, ice)
- Wear shoes or boots that provide good traction
- Replace smooth, worn out soles on footwear
- Throw out excessively worn footwear
- Only wear flip-flops or loose sandals when and where it is safe to do so
- Make sure that shoelaces are not too long, and are properly tied

Make accommodations as you age
- Keep your eyeglass prescription up to date, especially if you have bifocal lenses and/or eye disease

- Have your hearing checked and get a hearing aid if you need to
- Use your hearing aid if you have one
- If you get dizzy, be careful not to turn too quickly, and when getting out of bed, sit up first and give yourself a few moments to get your bearings before standing
- See your doctor if you often experience dizziness
- Be extra cautious when you are light-headed, have a head cold, allergies, or experience the side effects of drugs, alcohol, and medications
- Work with a physical therapist or other medical professional to purchase the appropriate walking aides and to learn safe procedures for using them
- Use appropriate walking aides, such as a canes, walkers, wheelchairs, or electric scooters, if you need them

What to do if you fall
- Stay calm and try to relax
- If you are out of harm's way, remain still for a short time to get over the initial shock of falling
- Assess whether you are injured before getting up
- If you think it is safe to get up, do it slowly and carefully
- If you don't think it is safe to get up, call out for help or use your phone to get help

What to do after you fall on a hazard if you are planning to contact an attorney
- Visit a hospital or doctor as soon as possible (ASAP)
- Take ample photos of the hazard, or have a friend or relative do so ASAP
- Talk to witnesses and get their names and phone numbers ASAP
- Write down notes of your memory of what you were doing before, during, and after you fell ASAP
- Get copies of accident reports
- Avoid admitting fault if you are contemplating a lawsuit

Takeaways
The next time I step into space - I will do it with grace

Falling hazards are commonplace in routes, at doorways, and on stairways. Counterintuitively, small irregularities can be hazardous because they are easily missed, while larger irregularities are often easier to recognize. We can minimize our risk of falling by learning how to spot hazards, and we can compensate for normal age-related changes to some extent by staying active, moving frequently, exercising, and keeping our minds sharp. We should all learn to practice cautious behavior, because whenever we walk anywhere, we assume some risk of falling. We can further reduce our risk of falling by minimizing distractions, taking responsibility for our own behavior, staying within our limits, and learning how to fall without getting injured.

Chapter 12

Stepping Forward: Advice for Professionals and Business Owners

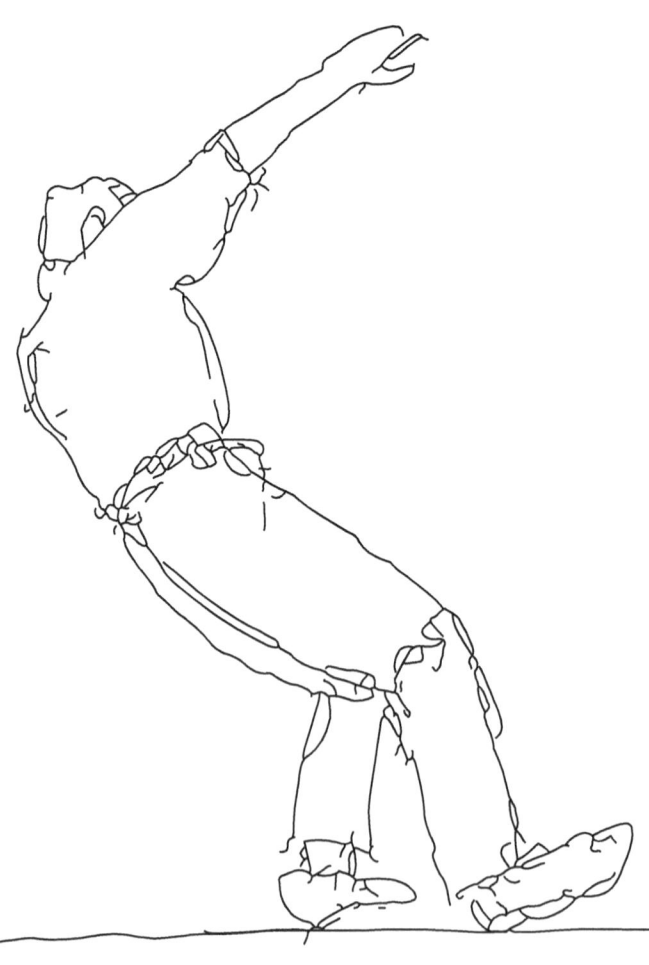

The costs of falls to our society, both financial and otherwise, is so enormous that it is for all practical purposes incalculable. Therefore, all of us have a responsibility to try to modify our walking and moving behavior and to do what we can to make the environment safer to reduce the possibility of falling.

State Authorities, Codes and Standards

An unfortunate reality is that many of the unsafe conditions described throughout this book have been known safety hazards for many years. Yet new buildings and sites are being constructed every day that do not follow common sense principles. As early as the 1970s there were research findings that should have been implemented in the form of stricter building codes. The Guidelines for Stair Safety research and report sponsored by the National Bureau of Standards in 1978 summarized a thorough review and analysis of stair safety and falls and environmental and human behavior issues that contribute to falls. Yet many of their findings have largely been ignored over the years rather than being adopted into standards and building codes. One recommendation in the report was to mark the edge of every tread in a stairway so that treads are more visually prominent. Although this would clearly reduce the number of falls, it is still not a requirement in most of the country, even though more than four decades have passed since the 1978 report was issued.

Since falls happen to everyone, and most of us will suffer a serious injury from a fall at some point in our lifetime, I recommend that building codes be updated to include additional common sense fall safety requirements.

Strict adherence to building codes should also be mandated for all buildings and sites everywhere. All states and territories should establish, if they have not done so already, procedures that quickly or automatically adopt the latest versions of the International Building Code (IBC), the International Residential Code (IRC), and/or the International Existing Building Code (IEBC). Building codes should be strictly enforced statewide, including every small community and rural area, even where there is no building code office, building official, or building inspector. Building codes should be supplemented with additional requirements to reduce the frequency of falls. For example, there should be a requirement to use slip-resistant paint when paints are used on parking lots, tapered curbs, and other locations. There should be clearly stated guidelines as to where painted warnings should be applied, and where they should not be applied, because when there are too many warnings, they lose their impact and tend to be ignored.

Code Officials, Inspectors, and Contractors

Building code officials and building and housing inspectors typically enforce minimum requirements but do not advise building owners to follow additional recommendations. I believe continuing education programs should educate building officials and inspectors to provide additional 'common sense' recommendations to contractors, home builders, and building owners. Since codes are minimum consensus documents, common sense recommendations are typically not included. For example, handrail color should contrast with wall color for greater visibility, and all stair treads should have contrasting strips on leading edges, even if these 'state of the art' practices are not yet code requirements. Code officials and inspectors should also be educated about falling hazards related to flooring materials, lighting, reflections and shadows, and should advise building owners about these issues. Since a high percentage of new buildings, additions, remodeled buildings, and site designs do not involve licensed architects or design professionals, getting this information to developers, property owners, and managers is essential to ensure that buildings and sites are as safe as possible and stand the test of time.

Building contractors also need to be educated to embrace the concept of making buildings and sites safe and inclusive for everyone. They have a responsibility to consult with professionals who have fall safety expertise to ensure designs incorporate safety features. This is especially true when there are no design professionals involved in projects.

Design Professionals

Just as building code officials and inspectors need to advise owners to construct beyond minimum standards, design professionals, including planners, architects, landscape architects, and interior designers, need to plan and design beyond minimums as well. When more inclusive designs, that make buildings and sites safer and easier to use by all people, are presented to clients, owners can be persuaded to incorporate those features. Many safety features add little or no cost to the overall cost of construction, if they are planned from the beginning. When owners realize that they will save on insurance cost over the long term because the number of expensive lawsuits will be reduced, many safety improvements can be easily justified.

When clients are shown safer designs from the beginning of the design process, they are often more likely to accept them. This needs to become a way of thinking for all design professionals. For example, building designs that have exterior grand stairways should not be shown to clients in the first place. Instead, site grading should be used to provide fully accessible entrances without ramps or stairs. This is not only more inclusive and safer for everyone, but it also saves owners maintenance costs, eventual ramp or stair rebuilding costs, and the worry, time, and financial costs of lawsuits after people fall.

Attorneys

People who fall and suffer injuries have a right to their day in court if they believe property owners are negligent. Our jury system works well, but the outcome for plaintiffs who fall is often short of people's expectations. Most attorneys I have had the pleasure to work with over the years have been competent and professional, but there have occasionally been situations that I prefer not to repeat. Attorneys can improve their chances of a successful outcome by providing enough information to experts and by informing experts of report submission deadlines and trial dates in a timely manner. They also need to allow experts adequate time to complete their research and fully develop their opinions. Defendants' attorneys need to resist badgering or harassing well qualified experts that are working for the plaintiff. It almost never works and leads to distrust and disrespect.

When representing plaintiffs, attorneys should always include demands that falling hazards are corrected by defendants. Defense attorneys should always advise their clients to make fall safety improvements, regardless of the conditions of a settlement or trial.

Expert Witnesses

Expert witnesses play an important role in providing the legal system with needed information and well-founded opinions. Both sides, plaintiffs and defendants, have a right to learn from experts' knowledge and opinions. Having well qualified experts involved in fall investigations can make a significant difference with respect to the outcome of a case. I have read reports and depositions of many experts and have made several observations regarding the common characteristics of good experts. Good experts are inquisitive, objective, honest, responsible, knowledgeable, thorough, and well qualified through their education, occupation, and/or experience. In their reports and testimony good experts do not slant, embellish, or diminish the truth. Experts who have worked for both the plaintiff and the defense tend to have understanding and empathy for both points of view. Good experts are fair, disciplined, measured, and reasonable. An important characteristic of a good expert is having the sensibility to admit what they know and what they don't know. Good experts also know how to empathize with individuals, how to relate to everyone, and how to speak in a layperson's language that is understandable by all people.

Shortcomings of expert witnesses who are not as effective are also worth noting. One problem is that some experts are too willing to venture out from their specific areas of expertise and offer opinions that are not well founded. I have also read many experts' reports that were couched in generalities but lacked specifics. They might state, for example, that there are numerous code violations, but they do not cite any specific ones. After reading some reports, it is very apparent that not enough time was spent doing research. Some experts use too much jargon, confusing the issues at hand, and making it difficult for people to understand what their point is. Sometimes this is done intentionally in an effort to impress or confuse people. It also happens when the expert does not adequately think through the circumstances of the falling event. Sometimes expert reports are filled with standardized, or boiler plate, one-size-fits-all narrative. However, each case is unique and although there may be similarities with other fall investigations, no two falling events are the same. Therefore, experts need to carefully and thoughtfully research the merits and circumstances of each case on an individual basis and prepare their reports accordingly. The process is not easy, and it always takes multiple drafts for me to explain everything in simple, straight forward language.

Restaurants and Lodging

Falls frequently occur both outside and inside restaurants and lodging facilities. This is at least partly because there are now so many restaurants and places of lodging, as new ones are spouting out of the ground like dandelions in the spring. Our country never seems to have enough of them.

While fall-preventative designs and details are more evident now than they were a few years ago, the restaurant and lodging industries need to go much further with this issue. As my wife can attest, almost every time we eat out or stay somewhere overnight, I observe and point out at least a couple of slip, trip, airstep, or other misstep hazards. Sometimes, but admittedly not often enough, I point them out to managers. Unfortunately, my suggestions usually get politely brushed aside and I see no changes or improvements when I return. Some managers are very receptive and appreciative, but most do not take my advice seriously until after someone falls.

I frequently observe several common problems at restaurants and places of lodging. Parking lots are often poorly designed with parking spaces that are too narrow and too tightly spaced. Drainage is often inadequate, resulting in puddling and ice forming in routes of travel. Curb stops for vehicle wheels are almost always tripping hazards. Curb ramps are frequently poorly designed and/or constructed without full compliance with ADA slope requirements. Tripping hazards are far too common and are frequently the result of differential settling due to inadequate drainage and/or inadequate compaction of soil, sand, and gravel under paved surfaces.

On the interior, buildings often have inappropriate flooring material near entrances that get slippery when wet. Poor quality or worn-out floor mats with rolled edges are also very common. Lighting inside entrances in restaurants and bars is often inadequate. Transition strips between flooring materials are often tripping hazards. Sunken or raised dining or lounge areas, where one or more steps are present, typically do not have adequate lighting or contrasting markings on the edges of platforms. Stairs usually do not have treads with edge markings, and/or proper handrails.

Other common fall safety issues include inadequate lighting throughout (often intentional to create a more intimate ambiance), reflections and shadows, busy and confusing floor patterns, single steps at booths without adequate lighting or easy to recognize edges, and overly crowded furniture arrangements.

Hotel and motel bathrooms are frequently designed so that everything fits into tight spaces with a minimum amount of floor space. Tight spaces can be hazardous when bathroom doors become obstacles, when toilets get placed too close to walls, cabinets, or bathtubs, and when there are no grab bars to hold onto. Tub-shower surfaces become slippery when wet and even slipperier when liquid soaps and shampoos are used. Many lodging chains only install grab bars where they are required in ADA accessible units. In my opinion every tub, tub-shower and shower and every toilet area in every lodging room should be equipped with appropriately placed grab bars that are securely anchored to withstand at least 250 lbs (1112 N) of force. Sometimes even that amount of resistance may not be enough. Towel bars should not be placed in any locations where people might grab onto them for support. If someone grabs onto a towel bar for support where there should be a grab bar, the towel bar will typically break loose from the wall and could result in an unnecessary fall and injury.

All lodging rooms should have lighted switches and/or night lights in the bathroom and other appropriate locations. Thermostats should have small LED lights and should be placed in easy-to-find locations at accessible heights, without furniture in front of them.

Owners, Managers, and Staff

Owners, managers, and maintenance staff of businesses, commercial establishments, and public institutions need to be proactive in order to halt our culture of falls. While it is true that there is plenty of blame to go around and that people who fall almost always contribute to the problem due to inattention or careless behavior, it is also true that unsafe conditions contributing to falls often get ignored by property owners until after people get injured, or after a lawsuit is filed.

A disproportionate number of falls seem to occur outside and inside small businesses. I sympathize with small-business owners who are struggling to pay rent and make a profit, but the safety of customers should always be front and center. Main street buildings often have sloped sidewalks that are not code-compliant because they have been modified incorrectly at entrances. Door thresholds are often tripping and/or airstep hazards because they are too high. Entry mats frequently have unsafe rolled edges that bunch up because the mats are of poor quality or are excessively worn. Overcrowding of displays and merchandise is commonplace. Single steps and uneven floors are common in old buildings and where two adjoining storefronts have been combined to form one retail space.

Owners or managers of small businesses need to inspect their premises frequently, be receptive to people who point out hazards, provide warning of unsafe conditions, and correct hazards before someone falls.

Recommendations for Owners, Managers, and Staff
Inspect exterior conditions
- Frequently inspect exterior site conditions including parking lots, curb ramps, exterior routes, sidewalks, exterior stairs, entrances and doors to identify slip, trip, and misstep hazards
- Regularly inspect parking lots and walking surfaces to identify potholes, poor drainage, and surface deterioration
- Identify heaved or dropped sections of concrete due to freeze-thaw cycles, settling, or tree roots
- Identify walking surfaces that are too smooth with inadequate slip resistance, and those that are too rough with excessive slip resistance
- Inspect walkways and routes of travel regularly for tripping hazards and excessive slopes
- Identify curb ramp and sidewalk intersections that are unsafe or do not comply fully with ADA Standards regarding slopes and/or side flares
- Inspect the edges of walks to ensure that they do not have hazardous drop offs and are level with the adjacent surfaces
- Identify large gaps between sections of paved walking surfaces that can catch shoes, canes, and walkers
- Observe drainage patterns over walks, curb ramps, drop off areas, entrances, and parking lots
- Identify objects including signs, tree branches, and building elements that protrude into routes

- Inspect the top and bottom of exterior stairways for dimensional uniformity
- Inspect all exterior and interior existing conditions to ensure full compliance with all applicable building codes, life safety codes, and ADA requirements

Inspect interior conditions
- Inspect all entrances, exits and doorways to identify unsafe tripping hazards at door thresholds
- Inspect entrance areas frequently for moisture and debris caused by the tracking in of snow, slush, sand, etc. on footwear
- Inspect floor mats for overall condition, secure grip, and flush edges
- Inspect stairs, floor surfaces, restrooms, and other public areas to identify slip, trip, and misstep hazards
- Inspect all flooring materials and transition strips between flooring materials to identify potential tripping or slipping hazards
- Measure lighting levels throughout interior spaces and evaluate lighting effectiveness, both quantitatively and qualitatively
- Identify distractions near stairs and raised floor areas
- Inspect the top and bottom of interior stairways for dimensional uniformity

Improve parking lots
- Ensure that the minimum standard parking space width is at least 9.5ft. (2.9m) [10ft. (3.0m) preferred]
- Do not install wheel stop tripping hazards in parking lots
- If wheel stops are present, eliminate them ASAP
- If wheel stops cannot be eliminated, ensure that they are properly located, anchored to the pavement, and painted a contrasting color
- Ensure that sidewalks bordering parking lots are wide enough (or install grass strips to separate parking lots from sidewalks) to maintain a safe accessible route width to prevent fronts of vehicles becoming obstacles and hazards for pedestrians and wheelchair users

- Ensure that all accessible parking spaces have access aisles
- Ensure that accessible parking spaces and access aisles do not slope more than 2% in any direction
- Use slip-resistant paint for parking lot striping and other pavement markings

Improve exterior routes
- Ensure that all sidewalk surfaces are firm, stable, and slip resistant
- Ensure that the running-slopes (slopes in the direction of travel) do not exceed 5% (1:20) in accessible routes
- Ensure that all sidewalks have cross-slopes (slopes perpendicular to the direction of travel) that do not exceed 2% (1:50)
- Ensure that all curb ramp and sidewalk intersections fully comply with ADA slope requirements
- Paint tripping hazards with a bright-color slip-resistant paint to provide warning and eliminate hazards as soon as possible

Improve curb ramps
- Use only curb ramp designs that follow all slope and dimensional requirements of the ADA Standards
- Do not bend, condense, warp, or stretch new curb ramps to fit existing conditions
- To reduce slipping and falling hazards, do not paint curb ramps or flared sides (tinting concrete flares is preferred)
- Construct curb ramp surfaces and flared sides surface with low slopes (1:14) or less
- Replace existing curb ramps when they do not fully comply with ADA Standards

Eliminate, or improve ramps
- Avoid installing ramps wherever possible by grading to provide fully accessible routes that do not exceed five percent running-slope and 2% cross-slope
- When ramps are necessary, construct them with the least slope possible (1:14 or less) and ensure that ramps fully comply with all ADA ramp requirements

- Ensure that transitions between ramps, landings, and sidewalks, are smooth and without tripping hazards

Improve entrances and doors
- Replace thresholds that are tripping hazards with safe, low profile thresholds
- Install high quality doors, door closers, and door hardware
- Install high quality automatic door openers where appropriate
- Place automatic door activators in appropriate locations that are not too close to doorways and are not in the direct path of travel
- Increase the length and width of vestibules to increase maneuvering space and reduce the chance of falling
- Install wider doors for easier access and increased safety
- Where possible, eliminate doors to increase access and safety

Improve flooring
- Install high quality, high traction flooring with good slip resistance
- Design corridors with appropriate natural and artificial lighting and window shading devices to minimize reflections and glare

Eliminate floor mats or choose high quality floor mats
- Eliminate loose floor mats, or replace them with integrated floor mats where possible
- Ensure floor mats are of high quality and are in good condition
- Ensure floor mats are heavy and large enough to stay in place
- Ensure floor mats have secure edging
- Clean floor mats frequently and remove contaminants such as dirt and sand
- Remove or replace worn-out floor mats

Improve stairway design and construction
- Modify or reconstruct stairways to comply with current building codes and the ADA Standards where possible and where appropriate

- Replace worn stair coverings before people slip, trip, or fall
- Install proper handrails with gripping profiles and extensions at the top and bottom of stairways where no handrails or insufficient handrails exist
- Ensure that the ends of handrails loop back, or to the wall, or to the floor, so they are not sleeve catchers
- Ensure that handrails contrast with wall colors so they are easy to see
- Ensure that all stairways are properly lit whenever the building is open
- Ensure that the top and bottom of all stairways are visually prominent and easy to recognize
- Ensure that all stair treads in a flight of stairs are the same solid color, and avoid visually confusing patterns
- To increase visibility, ensure that the leading edges of all stair treads have contrasting color
- Ensure that stair treads have adequate contrast with stair landings and floor surfaces at the top and bottom of stairs

Improve public restrooms
- Design and construct public restrooms without entrance doors while maintaining visual privacy to make access easier and falls less likely for everyone
- Design and construct public restrooms with continuous and level floor surfaces through doorways
- Choose appropriate plumbing fixtures to eliminate water splashing and spillage onto counters and floors
- Provide liquid-soap catch areas or locate liquid-soap dispensers over sinks to eliminate soap spillage on counters and floors
- Install slip resistant flooring
- Ensure that all floor surfaces are level
- Where floor drains are present, ensure that slopes to floor drains are gradual and minimal for drainage and that drain covers are level and are not slipping or tripping hazards
- In addition to providing wheelchair-accessible toilet stalls, provide ambulatory-accessible toilet stalls 3ft. (0.91m) wide,

higher toilet seats, grab bars on both sides, and out-swinging doors) in all rest rooms with two or more toilet stalls
- Install high-quality toilet partitions that are securely mounted and do not shake and move

Eliminate interior tripping hazards
- Ensure that carpeting is in good condition and is securely fastened without holes, rips, tears, or bunching
- Replace loose or bunched-up carpeting that cannot be securely fastened
- Ensure that transitions between flooring materials, such as from tile to carpet, are not tripping hazards and do not have vertical elevation changes over 0.25in. (6.4mm)
- Ensure that there is adequate lighting on all interior walking surfaces

Eliminate slipping hazards
- Ensure that floors have good slip resistance and are not too smooth
- Keep floor surfaces free of water, grease, and other liquids
- Ensure that floor areas that are prone to having water on them, including building entrances, restrooms, and areas near drinking fountains and sinks, are both slip resistant and not highly polished
- Keep entranceways dry and free of rain and snow that is tracked in by shoes and boots
- Use folding warning signs or warning cones where floors are wet, and remove as soon as floors are dry
- Use the appropriate slip-resistant floor cleaning and sealing products
- Use non-skid floor waxes on hard surface floors
- Refer to the fact sheet; Slip, Trips and Falls on Floors, National Safety Council, Revised Oct. 2016, for more recommendations

Improve exterior maintenance
- Identify and eliminate all tripping hazards in walking surfaces as soon as possible

- Level or replace sections of public sidewalks, or grind down small vertical changes in elevation, to eliminate tripping hazards to conform with ADA Standards
- Direct downspouts and drainpipes to discharge water into the ground or underneath sidewalks, rather than over sidewalks or plazas
- Raise the grade along walk edges where necessary to eliminate hazardous drop offs
- Keep exterior walking surfaces clear of obstacles, including toys, rocks, pebbles, leaves, twigs, and grass clippings
- Avoid using loose materials such as pebbles and mulch adjacent to walkways where they can easily spill over walking surfaces
- Ensure that stones, pebbles, and mulch in areas adjacent to sidewalks and parking lots are kept in place
- Sweep up remaining sand, salt, and ice melt chemicals after melting ice when walking surfaces are dry
- Eliminate or move hazardous signs, tree branches, or other obstacles that extend or protrude into routes from the side or above
- Seal cracks between landings and sidewalks, between driveways and sidewalks, and in sidewalks to prevent frost heave, settling, and tripping hazards

Improve interior maintenance
- Ensure that interior routes are kept clear of obstacles
- Eliminate or replace worn out or unsafe floor mats
- Do not over-wax or over-polish floors
- Train staff to identify and report spills and to clean them up as quickly as possible
- Offer incentives and awards to staff who identify and report falling hazards

Use warnings when and where appropriate
- Use warnings where appropriate, but always correct unsafe conditions ASAP
- Paint both top and vertical edges of tripping hazards with bright colored slip-resistant paint until hazards can be eliminated

- Paint both the top edge and vertical surfaces of tapered curbs adjacent to curb ramps with a bright color slip-resistant paint to provide visual cues where tripping hazards exist
- Place 'wet floor' signs and warnings on wet floors
- Remove 'wet floor' signs and warnings as soon as floors are dry

Takeaways
I controlled my fate by putting up a gate
We all fall short when it comes to our responsibility to be careful and to always 'be here now,' to prevent falls. A person's life can suddenly and dramatically change after suffering a fall. Improved observation skills will reduce the likelihood of falling. Warnings can be effective, but warnings are often missed by people, and warnings do not correct unsafe conditions. Hazards should always be eliminated as soon as possible. Each of us has a responsibility to recognize falling hazards and inform owners and managers about them since we all pay for falls in the form of lost wages, unnecessary medical and legal expenses, and higher health and property insurance rates.

Glossary

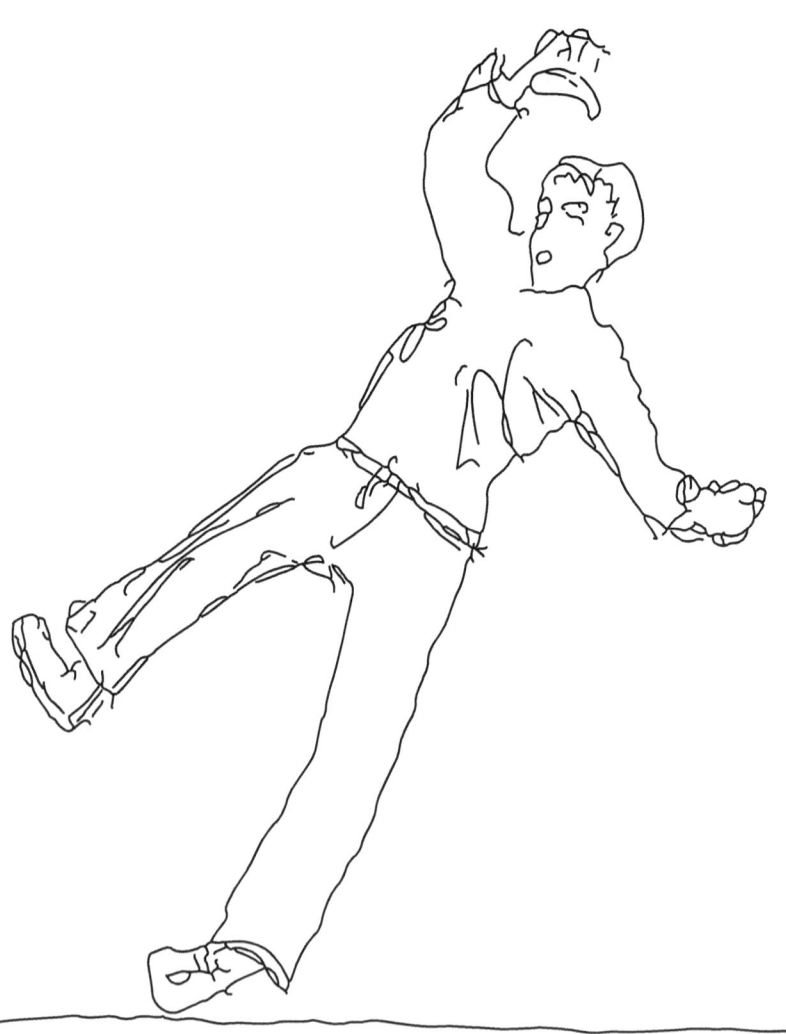

Below are the author's working definitions for the purpose of this publication. Please refer to other reliable sources for more complete or descriptive definitions.

Accessible entrance
> An entrance without steps or elevation changes that complies with the requirements of the ADA Standards.

Accessible parking
> Parking spaces that comply with the ADA Standards for accessible parking. Accessible parking spaces are reserved for people who meet ADA and state requirements as qualified persons with disabilities.

Accessible route
> A continuous unobstructed path of travel that complies with the requirements of the ADA Standards.

ADA Standards
> The Americans with Disabilities Act Standards for Accessible Design (ADASAD), more commonly known as the ADA Standards that are actually 'requirements' throughout the country, despite being titled as 'standards'

Airstep
> An unexpected step down or into a depression.

Building codes
: Government-adopted regulations that specify minimum requirements for design, construction, occupancy, and maintenance of buildings to protect the health, safety, and welfare of the public.

Coefficient of friction
: A measurement of the amount of resistance that a surface exerts on another surface. The coefficient of friction for flooring is accurately measured under controlled circumstances during flooring product development and testing. However, the coefficient of friction is difficult to accurately measure in the field after someone falls.

Construction industry standards
: Widely recognized standards by the design community and the construction industries (for example, "Walkway surfaces shall be firm, stable, and slip resistant.")

Construction joint
: A joint that separates sections of concrete walks and driveways that are poured separately at different times. Settling and freeze-thaw heaving cycles frequently result in tripping hazards at construction joints.

Control joint
: A line scored in concrete walks and driveways to facilitate cracks in those locations rather than other locations. Settling and freeze-thaw heaving cycles frequently result in tripping hazards forming at control joints.

Cross-slope
: The slope in a walking surface perpendicular to the direction of travel. A maximum of 2% cross-slope is permitted in accessible routes by the ADA Standards.

Curb ramp
: An accessible transition from an accessible route to a street, driveway, or parking lot that complies with specific ADA Standards.

Defendant(s)
: The person(s), or party(s) (building owner, company, business, etc.) who have a civil lawsuit filed against them by a plaintiff or plaintiffs.

Deposition
: Sworn testimony taken down in writing under oath. Typically, the answering of an attorney's questions to establish facts and opinions.

Detectable warning
: A textured warning on the surface of an accessible route or curb ramp, that meets the requirements of the ADA Standards, to alert people that they are about to cross a street or driveway.

Expert witness
: A qualified person with specialized expertise who provides professional opinions, typically in a written report, and/or testimony in a deposition and/or at trial.

Fall
: A fall occurs when a person's body suddenly descends freely under the force of gravity. Falls from a standing or walking position are most commonly the result from a trip, slip, unstable footing, airstep, over-step, under-step, or heel-scuff.

Grab bar
: A grab bar is a securely mounted bar that provides support and helps people maintain their balance and avoid falling. Grab bar dimensions, strength, and locations are specified for accessible restrooms, tubs, and showers in the ADA Standards.

Grandfathered code requirement
   A newer code requirement, not in an older version of the code, that is not enforceable because the building or site element in question was constructed before the newer code went into effect.

Guardrail
   A 42in. (1.1m) high (minimum) wall or railing, compliant with building code requirements, that is intended to prevent people from falling to a lower level.

Handrail
   A securely fastened railing used for grasping and support on stairways and ramps. Handrails should, but do not always, conform with specific building code requirements and/or ADA Standards regarding size, location, mounting height, and other parameters.

Hazard
   A source of potential injury to a person in the form of a condition in the physical environment that results in danger or risk, sometimes even when it is foreseeable.

Heel scuff
   Heel scuffs occur when people walking down short stair treads scrape the heels of their shoes on stair risers. Heel scuffs can result in falls.

Interrogatories
   Written questions that must be answered truthfully by either the plaintiff or defense to establish important facts.

Landing
   A flat level platform at the top or bottom of stairs, or between flights of stairs, or at the top or bottom of ramps, or between sloped sections of ramps, or inside or outside of doors and entrances.

Lighting Industry Standards
: Widely accepted standards for minimum lighting levels, and acceptable ranges for lighting levels, for specified areas and uses (for example, in public stairways).

Mediation
: An attempt to reach a mutually agreeable settlement between disputing parties (plaintiffs and defendants) with the help of an impartial mediator, typically to avoid a trial.

Misstep
: There are six types of missteps that have been identified and defined by Jake Pauls: trip, slip, unstable footing, airstep, over-step, and heel-scuff (Pauls, 2001)

Negligence
: Failure to exercise the degree of care that an ordinary person would exercise under the same circumstances.

Negligence per se
: When there is a specific violation of a specific code or ordinance.

Nosing
: The leading edge of a stair tread. In residential stairs the nosing typically projects approximately 0.75in. (19.1mm) over the riser below it. Projecting nosing can be hazardous toe catchers.

Overstep
: An over-step occurs when part of a person's foot is placed too far forward on a stair tread, a single step, or an edge of a landing.

Plaintiff
: The person (typically the person that falls) who files a suit in a court of law to seek a remedy and/or financial compensation.

Riser
: The vertical part of a single stair.

Running slope
: The slope in the direction of travel. The ADA Standards established maximum running slopes for accessible routes, curb ramps, and ramps.

Side flare
: A side flare is a triangular shaped section of surface on a curb ramp that should fully comply with the slope requirements of the ADA Standards. Side flares can be hazardous when they have excessive slopes or when they do not fully comply with ADA Standards.

Slip
: A slip happens when a person's foot or footwear loses traction due to an unexpected reduction in friction.

Spalling
: The breaking up and deterioration of a brick, tile, concrete, or asphalt walking surface after water migrates into cracks, freezes and expands.

Stair
: The International Building Code (IBC) defines a stair as, "A change in elevation, consisting of one or more risers."

Stair flight (or flight of stairs)
: A set of stairs between landings in a stairway (for example, if a stairway has one intermediate landing, the stairway has two flights of stairs).

Stairway
: A stairway includes stairs, landings, and handrails.

Tapered curb
: A curb that tapers over a length from a normal curb height at one end to a smooth transition of surfaces at the other end. A tapered curb typically occurs at curb ramps where side-flares are present.

Threshold
: A plastic, wood or metal transition strip at the bottom of a door or doorway. High, or severely sloped thresholds are often tripping hazards. Low profile thresholds are preferred.

Tread
: The horizontal part of a single stair.

Trip
: A trip typically happens when a person stubs the toe of their footwear on an unexpected projection in the walking surface.

Unstable footing
: A fall results from unstable footing when a person's foot does not make adequate contact with a surface. It typically occurs at raised edges or ends of walks, or when a person encounters an unexpected deviation, depression, or slope in a walking surface.

Warning
: A warning of a fall hazard can take the form of; 1) painting the top and vertical edges of a tripping hazard a bright color to make it more visible, 2) barricading off an area, 3) placing warning cones or folding warning signs over and/or near a hazard, or 4) signs posted on walls or doorways. Warnings should be considered as temporary measures and falling hazards should be eliminated as soon as possible.

References and Readings

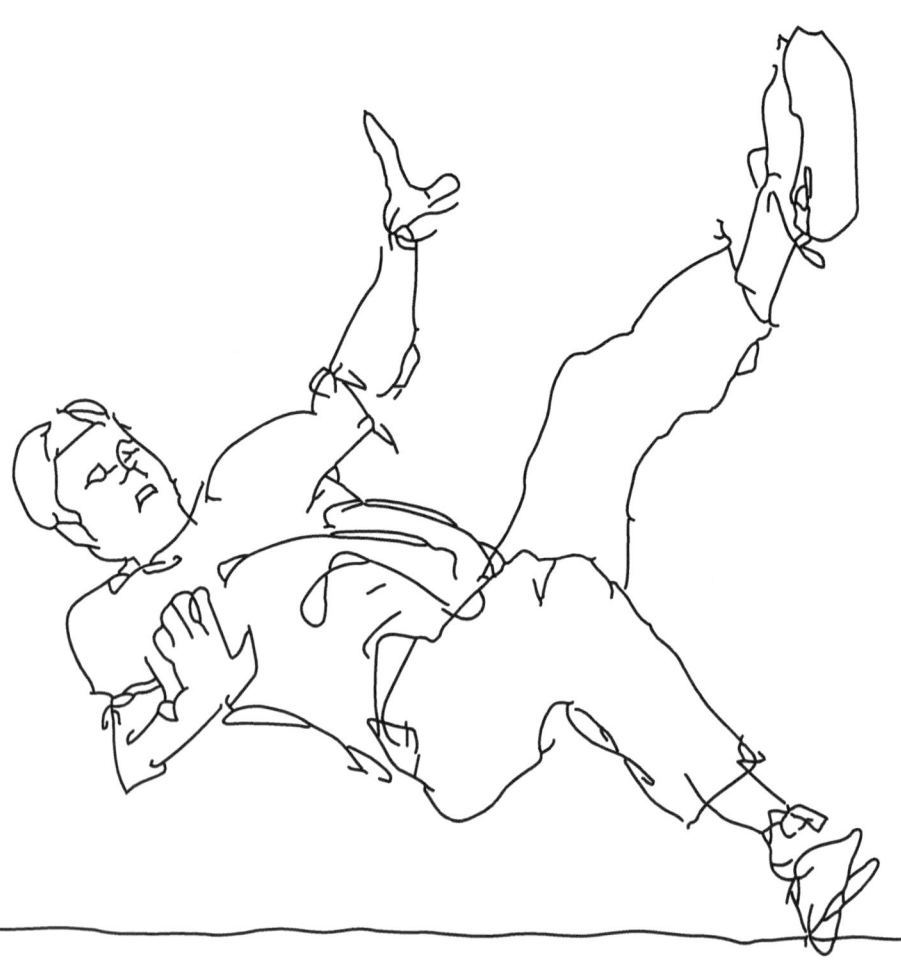

A Guide for Maintaining Pedestrian Facilities for Enhanced Safety, USDOT, Federal Highway Commission

Archea, J., Collins, B.L. & Stahl, F. I., *Guidelines for stair safety,* NBS Building Science Series 120, U.S. Department of Commerce National Bureau of Standards, Washington, 1979

Bakken, Cohen, Abele, Hyde, and LaRue, *Slips, Trips, Missteps and Their Consequences,* Second Edition, Lawyers and Judges Publishing Co., 2007

Boyd, Robynne, *Do People Only Use 10 Percent of Their Brains?* in Scientific American, February 7, 2008

Brody, Jane E., *Growing Older, and Adjusting to the Dark,* in New York Times, March 13, 2007

Carson, Archea, Margulis, *Safety on Stairs,* NBS Building Science Series 108, U.S. Department of Commerce National Bureau of Standards, Washington, 1978

Casner, Steve, *Careful, A User's Guide to Our Injury-Prone Minds,* Riverhead Books, 2017

Cohen, Harvey H., and Pauls, Jake, *Warning and Markings for Stairways and Pedestrian Terrain*, Chapter 57 in Handbook of Warnings, edited by Michael S. Wogalter, Lawrence Erlbaum Associates, 2006

Cohen, Joseph, LaRue, Cindy A., and Cohen, H. Harvey, *Stairway Falls, an ergonomics analysis of 80 cases*, in Profession Safety, January 2009

Di Pilla, Steven, *Slip, Trip, and Fall Prevention, A Practical Handbook*, CRC Press, 2010

Fair Housing Design Manual, a free manual that includes guidance for the design and construction of housing to comply with the Fair Housing Act
https://www.huduser.gov/portal/publications/destech/fairhousing.html

Fruin, John J., *Pedestrian Planning and Design*, Revised Edition, Elevator World, Inc., 1987

Hallinan, Joseph T., *Why We Make Mistakes*, Broadway Books, New York, 2009

Hsiao, Hongwei, editor, *Fall Prevention and Protection, Principles, Guidelines, and Practices*, CRC Press, 2017

Hutton, J. Thomas, M.D., Ph.D., *Preventing Falls, A Defensive Approach*, Promestheus Books, 2000

Johnson, Fred M., Ph.D., *Slips and Falls, A New Approach to Friction Measurements*, Lawyers and Judges Publishing Co., 2008

Jolly, David N., *The Slip and Fall Handbook*, Outskirts Press, 2013

Jones, Michael A., *Accessibility Standards Illustrated*, published by the State of Illinois, 1978

Kendzior, Russell J., Falls Aren't Funny, America's Multi-Billion-Dollar Slip-and-Fall Crisis, Scarecrow Press, Inc., 2010

Mack, Arien and Rock, Irvine, Inattentional Blindness, MIT Press, 1998

Marletta, William, Trip, Slip, and Fall Protection, Chapter 12, in The Work Environment, Volume One, Occupational Health Fundamentals, Doan J. Hansen, Editor, Lewis Publishers, 1991

Murphy, Kate, The Right Way to Fall, in The New York Times, January 24, 2017

Nonfatal Fall-Related Injuries Associated with Dogs and Cats, United States, 2001-2006, Centers for Disease Control (cdc.gov)

Noy, Ian Y. and Karwoski, Waldemar, editors, Handbook of Human Factors in Litigation, Chapter 38, Human Factors Terminology, CRC Press, 2005

O'Connor, Anahad, Stairs at Home Remain a Childhood Hazard, New York Times, March 12, 2012

O'Rahilly, M.D., Ronan, Muller, Dr., Fabriola, Carpenter, Ph.D., Stanley, and Swenson, M.D., Rand, Basis Human Anatomy, 2004

Osterberg, Dr. Arvid E., Access for Everyone, A Guide to the Accessibility of Buildings and Sites with references to ADASAD, Third Edition, published by Facilities Planning & Management, Iowa State University 2010
    For a free digital download, go to https://www.fpm.iastate.edu/capital_projects/standards_procedures.asp

Osterberg, Dr. Arvid E., Preventing Falls in Housing Environments, presented at the Annual Conference on The Sociology of Housing, St. Paul, MN, 1993

Pauls, Jake, *Are Functional Handrails Within Our Grasp?* in *The Building Official and Code Administrator*, March/April 1991

Pauls, Jake, *Life Safety Standards and Guidelines Focused on Stairways*, Chapter 23 in *Universal Design Handbook*, Wolfgang F.E. Preiser and Elaine Ostroff, editors, McGraw-Hill, 2001

Pauls, Jake, CPE, *Representation of the Elderly in Premises Liability Cases with a Focus on Falls*, in Reference Materials, Vol. II, Convention of the Association of Trial Lawyers of America, Chicago, 2000

Seniorology: The Ultimate Guide to Keep Seniors Safe from Slips, Trips, and Falls, Kindle Edition, Sold by Amazon Digital Services, LLC., 2017

Sinnott, Ralph, *Safety and Security in Building Design*, Van Nostrand Reinhold Co., 1985

Standard Practice for Walkway Surfaces, American Society for Testing and Materials (ASTM) (Designation: F 1637 – 95)

The People's Law Dictionary, Gerald N. Hill and Kathleen Thompson Hill, Barns and Noble Books, New York, 2002

Templer, John, *The Staircase: Studies of Hazards, Falls, and Safer Design*, MIT Press, Cambridge, Mass, 1992

Tideiksaar, Rein, *Falls in Older People, Prevention and Management*, Fourth Edition, Health Professions Press, 2010

Turnbow, Charles E., *Slip and Fall Practice*, Second Edition, James Publishing, 1997

Zorn, Eric, *An important reminder about head injuries in the death of Walter Jacobson's wife*, in the Chicago Tribune, 5/3/2019

Fact Sheets and Short Guides

Accessible Sidewalks and Street Crossings, an informational guide, U.S. Department of Transportation, Federal Highway Administration

Designing Sidewalks and Trails for Access, U.S. Department of Transportation, Federal Highway Administration

Falls Fact Sheet, World Health Organization, 2018

Fall Prevention Fact Sheet, National Council on Aging, 2012

Injury Facts, 2015 Edition, National Safety Council

Important Facts about Falls, Centers for Disease Control and Prevention

Preventing Falls on Stairs, Canada Mortgage and Housing Corporation

A Guide for Maintaining Pedestrian Facilities for Enhanced Safety, U.S. Department of Transportation, Federal Highway Administration

Slip, Trip, and Fall Prevention for Healthcare Workers, Department of Health and Human Services, Centers for Disease Control and Prevention, National Institute for Occupational Safety and Health

Stairway Safety; a pdf presentation, Auburn University

World Health Organization
    www.who.int/mediacentre/factsheets/fs344/en/

Website Resources

American Association of Retired People - aarp.org
Access Board - access-board.gov
ADA National Network - adata.org
Canada Safety Council - canadasafetycouncil.org
Center for Disease Control and Prevention (CDC) - cdc.gov
National Floor Safety Institute - nfsi.org
National Safety Council - ncs.org
Visitability - visitability.org

About the Author

Dr. Arvid Osterberg is University Professor at Iowa State University, where he teaches graduate courses on inclusive design and historic preservation in the Department of Architecture. During his 43+ years at ISU, he has taught students to prioritize accessibility and safety. Arvid has consulted with attorneys on fall investigations throughout his career. He is a registered architect and holds two degrees in architecture from the University of Illinois and a doctorate in architecture from the University of Michigan.

Index

B

Balance 14, 20, 28, 30, 32, 67, 69, 76, 79, 82, 83, 89, 96, 100, 107, 108, 123, 157, 158, 160-163, 166, 170, 171, 173, 181, 184-186, 209
Basement stairs 19, 131, 136
Bathroom 21, 57-60, 128, 129, 135, 197
Battle of the Experts 148
Benign Paroxysmal Positional Vertigo (BPPV) 160
Black ice 28, 33, 82, 156, 181, 184
Blame 9, 33, 53, 69, 142, 151, 166, 168, 169, 197
Booth 101-103
Building code 36, 37, 45, 47, 48, 55-58, 60, 87, 88, 90, 102, 107, 108, 110-113, 115-118, 132, 174, 192, 193, 210
Building code violation 90
Burden of proof 58, 113, 148

A

Accessible entrance 77
Accessible parking 75-77, 200, 207
Accessible route 75-78, 97, 199, 209
ADA Standards 38, 47, 49, 52, 53, 60, 70, 72, 73, 75-78, 87, 88, 95, 97, 101, 107, 112, 115, 116, 151, 170, 171, 173, 174, 181, 182, 198, 200, 201, 204, 207, 208, 209, 210, 212
Airstep 28, 29, 66, 74, 75, 82, 87, 92, 102, 110, 121, 122, 166, 170, 175, 182, 196, 197, 209, 211
Attorney 9, 43, 44, 46-48, 50, 51, 53, 54, 56-59, 69, 70, 72, 74-80, 87, 91, 96-98, 100, 102, 110-117, 121, 132, 133, 141-144, 146, 148-150, 152, 187, 209
Awareness 21, 22, 39, 63, 103, 161, 169, 170, 174-177, 184

C

Cane 85, 163
Carpeting 20, 21, 97, 100, 101, 113, 114, 135, 136, 138, 156, 203
Cats 163, 217
Caution 79, 96, 118, 124, 160, 178, 183, 184
Center of gravity 48, 69, 82, 83, 117, 157, 163
Church 112, 113, 155
Clear ice 181
Code violation 90, 117, 149
Coefficient of friction 208
Common sense 36, 54, 128, 130, 157, 191, 192
Comparative negligence 145, 146
Compensation 9, 43, 49, 51, 53, 55, 70, 73, 80, 97, 111, 113, 115, 122, 132, 142-147, 150, 211
Complacency 130

Concussion 16, 25, 26, 57, 87, 106, 132, 156
Construction industry standards 36, 208
Construction joint 208
Control joint 66, 70
Cross-slope 17, 45, 51-53, 62, 78, 175, 200, 208
Curb ramp 72, 73, 156, 171, 198, 200, 209, 212

D

Defendant 43, 90, 113, 133, 143, 145
Deposition 70, 74, 77, 79, 86, 87, 110, 114, 142, 146, 209
Descending 32, 54, 107, 108, 112, 119, 164, 171
Design 9, 10, 15, 21, 36-38, 44, 52, 72, 73, 76, 78, 102, 106, 118, 123, 128, 130, 151, 171, 173, 193, 201, 208, 216
Detectable warning 156
Dishwasher door 32
Distracting 118, 158, 165
Distraction 164, 176, 177
Dizziness 106, 123, 160, 162, 187
Dogs 32, 68, 163, 164
Dogs and cats 163
Door 25, 29, 31, 32, 45, 46, 48, 50, 51, 54-59, 61, 71, 72, 86-92, 110, 114, 115, 121, 122, 128, 132, 134, 178, 199, 201, 213
Doorway 17-19, 46, 56, 58, 61, 62, 85-88, 91, 97, 110, 170, 213
Driveway 17, 31, 55, 133, 209

E

Electric scooter 17, 51-53, 61, 62
Elevators 121, 123, 124
Entrance 47, 55, 56, 71, 72-77, 86, 89, 128, 129, 171, 184, 199, 202, 207
Escalator 121, 123
Expert witness 45, 68, 146, 147, 148

F

Fall 9, 13-21, 26-35, 39, 43-47, 50, 51, 53-58, 60-62, 66, 67, 69, 78, 79, 81, 85-89, 91, 95, 100-103, 106-116, 121, 122, 127, 128, 130, 133, 139, 141-144, 148, 150-152, 157-161, 163, 165, 166, 167, 169, 170, 176, 179, 180, 183, 185, 187, 188, 192-197, 202, 205, 209, 213
Falling 10, 13-15, 18, 21, 22, 25, 27, 28, 30, 31, 34-36, 40, 43, 47, 48, 54, 57, 60, 62, 63, 65, 67-69, 75, 78, 80, 81, 83, 86, 90, 92, 95, 96, 106-108, 118, 122-124, 129-131, 133, 139, 141, 147, 148, 150-152, 155-163, 165-167, 169, 170, 172, 173, 175, 176, 178, 179, 183-185, 187, 188, 191, 192, 194, 195, 200, 201, 204, 205, 209, 210, 213
Fear of falling 130, 155, 156, 161
Financial compensation 9, 43, 51, 53, 55, 70, 73, 80, 97, 111, 113, 115, 122, 132, 144, 145, 147, 211
Flip-flops 142, 179, 186
Floor 17, 18, 20, 21, 28, 32, 38, 54, 58, 59, 86, 87, 89, 90, 95-103, 108-111, 114, 116, 121, 122, 127-130, 133-135, 138, 142, 159, 166, 172, 176-178, 182, 185, 196, 199, 201-205
Flooring 38, 39, 95, 97, 103, 108, 129, 133, 135, 150, 171, 192, 196, 199, 201-203, 208

223

Floor mat 98, 99
Foot-candle 50, 87, 110, 114
Footwear 28, 39, 68, 81, 95, 103, 131, 142, 158, 169, 179, 186, 199, 212, 213
Force of gravity 14, 209
Fraud 150
Freeze-thaw 180, 181, 198, 208
Friction 28, 39, 208, 212
Funeral home 113, 114
Funny 31, 32

G

Gait 157, 162
Garage doors 32, 185
Glare 68, 136, 138, 139, 201
Glaucoma 162
Grab bar 21, 59-62, 129, 130, 197, 209
Grandfathered 117
Grass 31, 47, 62, 73, 80-82, 182, 183, 199, 204
Grass covered 183
Gripping profile 107, 113, 116, 138
Guardrail 47, 48, 53, 89, 90, 116, 117

H

Handrail 19, 20, 43, 54, 55, 62, 74, 77, 89, 90, 107, 112-116, 119, 131, 132, 136, 166, 192
Hazard 15-17, 33, 46, 47, 54, 62, 66-68, 70-75, 86, 88, 97, 98, 101, 109, 116, 131, 141, 149-151, 157, 166, 169, 172, 175, 176, 181, 182, 184, 187, 213
Heel-scuff 28, 29, 108, 209, 211
Home 16, 27, 28, 35, 48-50, 62, 71, 113, 114, 127-130, 133, 136, 139, 157, 162, 164, 178, 192
Homeowner 79, 127, 132, 133
Hotel 58-60, 171

I

Industry standards 36, 39, 49, 70, 98, 107, 146, 148, 151, 208
Information overload 175
Interrogatories 44, 146

K

Kitchen 25, 57, 129, 132, 135

L

Landing 22, 31, 45, 46, 51, 55-58, 62, 77, 87, 89, 90, 106, 132, 159, 211, 212
Lawsuit 43, 59, 91, 97, 106, 112, 132, 152, 187, 197, 209
Lighting 33, 37, 43, 44, 50, 51, 55, 58, 62, 68, 81, 85, 87, 100-102, 106, 110-114, 123, 127, 135, 137, 138, 159, 161, 165, 174, 176, 178, 179, 181, 183, 186, 192, 196, 199, 201, 203, 211
Lighting Industry Standards 211
Lodging 60, 195, 196, 197

M

Macular degeneration 162
Maintain 46, 60, 63, 67, 69, 70, 76, 87, 106, 107, 147, 157, 160, 161, 163, 170, 181, 184, 186, 199, 209
Manager 75, 100, 142, 144
Mediation 73, 144
Misstep 28, 107, 108, 176, 196, 198, 199
Motel 60, 196
Moving Devices 5, 120, 121, 123
Moving walkway 122, 123
Multi-tasking 168, 177

N

Negligence 34, 48, 50, 90, 111-113, 142-146, 152
Negligence per se 48, 90, 111, 113
Negligent 34, 49, 51, 53, 54, 58, 71, 81, 101, 106, 111, 113, 114, 122, 127, 133, 142, 143, 145, 146, 152, 194
Neurological disorders 162
Nosing 211

O

Observation 9, 15, 21, 31, 44, 81, 174, 184, 205
Observe 21, 22, 66, 68, 82, 95, 168, 171, 174-176, 180, 183, 195, 196
Observing 65, 167, 174, 175
Obstacle 28, 67, 68, 137
Over-step 19, 20, 28, 29, 105, 108, 118, 119, 209, 211
Owner 33, 34, 39, 43, 45-51, 53-57, 60-62, 70-72, 74-81, 90, 99, 101, 111, 112, 115, 123, 127, 128, 142, 144, 146, 169, 209

P

Pets 32, 68, 164
Plaintiff 43-45, 47, 49, 53, 57, 58, 62, 73, 80, 98, 99, 101, 113, 132, 133, 143-150, 152, 169, 194, 209, 210
Pothole 29, 75, 76, 181
Public building 127, 166

R

Railing 47, 55, 90, 110, 116, 119, 210
Raised booth 103
Ramp 52, 72, 73, 77, 88, 89, 100, 156, 171, 193, 198, 200, 209, 212

Rebuttal 150
Responsibility 13, 22, 39, 49, 60, 62, 70, 78, 99, 111, 118, 165, 167-169, 179, 188, 191, 193, 205
Restaurant 15, 18, 19, 46, 47, 69, 70, 86-88, 101, 102, 171, 178, 195
Restroom 97, 101, 110, 111, 116, 178
Riser 29, 45, 106, 108, 109, 112, 119, 151, 166, 170, 171, 174, 181, 183, 211
Risk 9, 35, 69, 80, 81, 118, 119, 123, 131, 133, 139, 144, 162, 165-167, 169, 170, 172, 183, 184, 188, 210
Risk threshold 170
Risky 31, 65, 131, 146, 166, 184
Running-slope 77, 200

S

Safety 10, 27, 36-38, 44, 49-51, 55, 60, 68, 87, 88, 91, 101, 102, 107-109, 111, 112, 115, 118, 128-130, 133, 137-139, 148, 168, 174, 176, 183, 191-194, 196, 197, 199, 201, 208, 215
Segway 79, 80
Sensory overload 177, 178
Settlement 48, 58, 73, 88, 90, 98, 113, 122, 146, 148, 168, 194, 211
Side flare 212
Sidewalk 14-17, 22, 28, 29, 31, 33, 43, 45, 46, 50-54, 61, 62, 65-74, 77-80, 82, 83, 87, 112, 134, 142, 143, 155, 164, 171, 175, 176, 180-184, 198, 200
Single step 29, 72, 74, 75, 85, 88, 181, 211
Site inspection 44-47, 51, 53, 57, 59, 69, 78, 91, 97, 98, 148
Slip 16, 18, 21, 22, 28, 30, 38, 39, 59, 60, 66, 75, 81, 95, 99, 103, 129, 133, 135, 138, 139, 144, 179,

181, 185, 186, 192, 196, 198-205, 208, 209, 211, 212
Slipping 16, 28, 31, 39, 60, 62, 80, 95, 96, 129, 135, 166, 178, 199, 200, 202, 203
Slip resistance 28, 38, 39, 59, 135, 138, 179, 186, 198, 201, 203
Spalling 48, 49
Stair 19, 20, 29, 32, 45, 54, 55, 106-109, 112, 113, 118, 127, 131-133, 136-139, 166, 171, 172, 174, 183, 184, 191-193, 202, 210-213, 215
Stair flight (or flight of stairs) 212
Stairway 19, 20, 32, 51, 54-58, 61, 62, 89, 90, 105-116, 118, 119, 131, 132, 137-139, 151, 156, 158, 164-167, 170-174, 177, 183, 191, 201, 212
Steep stairway 108, 113, 119, 131
Surveillance video 39, 95, 96, 121, 150

T

Tai Chi 160
Tapered curb 71, 72, 213
Threshold 17, 46, 47, 61, 62, 85-89, 170
Towel bar 59, 60, 62, 130, 197
Traumatic brain injury 25, 110, 112, 121, 122, 132
Tread 19, 29, 106, 108, 113, 136, 151, 174, 191, 211
Trial 46-49, 51, 53-55, 57, 58, 60, 70, 71, 73, 74, 76-80, 87-90, 96-99, 101, 111-117, 122, 123, 132, 133, 142, 144, 146, 147, 150, 152, 169, 194, 209, 211
Trip 14, 16, 17, 22, 28, 32, 66, 68, 69, 71, 81, 83, 92, 103, 108, 109, 135, 151, 155, 166, 174, 176, 186, 196, 198, 199, 202, 209, 211, 213

Tripping hazard 15, 16, 46, 47, 66-68, 70-74, 86, 97, 98, 141, 150, 151, 157, 175, 176, 181, 184, 213
Tub-shower 21, 58-62, 197

U

Under-step 20, 28, 29, 108, 209
Unsafe 29, 33, 34, 45-47, 49-51, 53-55, 57, 58, 60, 70-74, 78-81, 86, 88-91, 99-102, 106, 107, 109-118, 130-132, 134, 146-148, 150, 167, 169, 173, 175-177, 179, 191, 197-199, 204, 205
Unsafe behavior 175
Unsafe conditions 29, 45, 54, 57, 73, 78, 79, 86, 89, 112, 113, 116, 118, 130, 132, 147, 169, 191, 197, 198, 204, 205
Unstable footing 28, 66, 76-78, 82, 157, 171, 209, 211, 213

V

Vertigo 160
Vision 15, 33, 36, 38, 67, 69, 74, 81, 102, 105, 119, 122, 161-163, 167, 175, 176, 182, 186
Visitability 129, 220

W

Walker 47, 62, 85, 156, 163
Walking 14, 16, 18, 19, 28, 29, 32, 34, 38, 39, 43, 46, 50-52, 65-69, 73-75, 79, 80, 82, 83, 85, 86, 88, 89, 91, 95-97, 106, 108, 109, 111, 114, 115, 118, 128, 131, 134, 135, 155-158, 162-168, 170-177, 180, 181, 183-187, 191, 198, 203, 204, 208-210, 212, 213

Warning 14, 33, 46, 49, 70, 74, 78, 86,
	88, 96, 122, 146, 156, 176, 177,
	198, 200, 203, 209, 213
Wheelchair 50-52, 61, 62, 75, 85, 86,
	88, 97, 100, 173, 199, 202
Wheel stops 81, 199
Witness 45, 68, 91, 146-148, 209

Y

YouTube 31, 60

www.ingramcontent.com/pod-product-compliance
Lightning Source LLC
Chambersburg PA
CBHW051540020426
42333CB00016B/2021